HEMIFACIAL SPASM
These are our stories

Kimberly P. Robinson

Copyright: 2020 by Kimberly P. Robinson
All rights reserved.

CONTRIBUTORS

I would like to personally thank each of the following individuals for being brave enough to contribute the story of their personal journey to this book. - Kim Robinson

Trixie
Susan Nofi
Shirl Boatman
Sharina Samarista
Joe Pane
Denise Starkey
Darla OLeary
Jenny Sander
Jane Winlow
Kim Puckett
Fabiola Teresa
Karrie Ward
Brenda Kyne
Louise Walker
Samudhyatha Bhat
Angela Bond
Cindy Teta

Also, a very special thank you to Dr. Ashley Robinson for her assistance with this project, including cover photography.

HEMIFACIAL SPASM
THESE ARE OUR STORIES

Kimberly P. Robinson

This book is a compilation of true stories from actual Hemifacial Spasm sufferers across the world. Each story is written differently, in their own words, describing their journey with this difficult and often debilitating condition. You will not only read accounts of their medical experiences with Hemifacial Spasm, but you will also hear about their emotional experiences. For various reasons, hospital and doctors' names have been omitted from the stories. As you will see, many individuals affected by this condition have found resolution; however, there are still others who continue to suffer on a daily basis. It is my hope that, one day, each person will find relief from this horrible condition called Hemifacial Spasm.

Individual	Location	Current Age	Estimated Age of Onset	Number of MVD Surgeries	Additional Treatments (both successful and unsuccessful listed)	Most Successful HFS Treatment	Current HFS Status	Page
Kimberly Robinson	North Carolina, USA	54	49	1	Botox, Anti-Seizure Meds., Muscle Relaxers, Marinol, Clonazepam, Pain Killers, Xidra, Restastis, Antibiotics, Bio-Feedback, Prednisone Packs, Steroid Infusions	MVD (30% improvement) Steroid Infusions (50% improvement- short lived)	Present, but slightly reduced.	6
Trixie	Manila, Philippines	42	31	2	Botox, Zen meditation, Acupuncture, Yoga, Taiichi, and Functional Medicine	MVD	Present, but greatly reduced	16
Susan Nofi	Massachusetts, USA	73	36	3	Medications, including a Muscle Relaxant, and Psychotherapy	MVD	Spasm free but noticeable weakness on the MVD side	19
Shirl Boatman	Illinois, USA	59	50	0	Botox	None	Present	22
Sharina Samarista	Camarines Sur, Philippines	30	20	1	Botox, Rivotril	MVD	Almost 100% spasm-free	25
Joe Pane	Melbourne, Australia	51	46	2	Botox, Tegretol	Botox	Present	27
Denise Starkey	United Kingdom	57	48	1	Botox	MVD	Spasm free	29
Darla OLeary	New Jersey, USA	67	60	1	Botox, Acupuncture, Anti-seizure drug	Botox	Present, but reduced	30
Jenny Sander	Queensland, Australia	62	45	1	Rivotril	MVD	Spasm free	32
Jane Winlow	United Kingdom	36	33	2	Botox, No Caffeine	MVD	Present, but greatly reduced	40
Kim Puckett	Auckland, New Zealand	46	36	2	Botox	MVD	Almost 100% spasm-free	44
Fabiola Teresa	Aguascalientes, Ags. Mexico	41	29	2	Homeopathy, Acupuncture, Naturopathic Medicine, Botox, Clonazepam, Magnesium Valproate, Baclofen, Carbamazepine, Psychological Therapies	MVD	Present, but slight improvement	47

Individual	Location	Current Age	Estimated Age of Onset	Number of MVD Surgeries	Additional Treatments (both successful and unsuccessful listed)	Most Successful HFS Treatment	Current HFS Status	Page
Karrie Ward	Oklahoma, USA	60	49	2	Botox, Antibiotics, Neurontin, Lyrica, Carbamazepine, Klonopin, Aripiprazole, Prednisone, Elavil, Baclofen	MVD	Spasm free	50
Brenda Kyne	Northern California, USA	58	56	2	Botox, Magnesium L-Threonate	MVD	Spasm free	52
Louise Walker	England	40	28	2	Botox, Alternative Therapies	MVD	Bi-lateral (Left side spasms and Right side mostly spasm free)	54
Samudhyatha Bhat	Bangalore, India	33	29	1	B12, Tegretol, Ayurvedic Meds.	MVD	Spasm free	58
Angela Bond	UK	69	54	1	Botox, Carbamazepine	MVD	Spasm free	59
Cindy Teta	Pennsylvania, USA	64	55	1	None	Unknown at this time	Present	67
Glossary								69

Kimberly Robinson

My name is Kimberly Robinson. I'm a 54-year-old female from North Carolina, USA. I have left sided Hemifacial Spasms and secondary blepharospasms. This is my story.

Before you proceed, I want to warn you. I'm writing the story of my Hemifacial Spasm journey from the heart. Don't expect it to be polished or "sugar coated" because, for me, it's been anything but that. I'm a private person by nature so this is not an easy journey for me to share publicly, mainly because it is so emotionally painful. Or, maybe I'm even somewhat embarrassed to let the world "in" to see my raw vulnerability. I've always taken pride in being a strong woman, but at times, especially when I'm alone, I feel I have lost that identity. I do want to make it clear that I'm not doing this for me. The last thing I want is pity and I believe that a lot of us with this condition feel this way. What I do want is awareness, understanding and compassion for all of us out there who are suffering from this debilitating condition. If at least one story in this book that I have compiled can help someone, then my mission has been accomplished.

Most mornings I wake up early, sometimes as early as 5:00 a.m. Reality usually kicks in and, on my worst days, the tears can come easy. I have learned to become a silent crier so that I don't wake my husband. It's going on six years now of suffering. The spasms (and most days the pain) begin immediately. In a constant struggle to open my eyes, I reach over to start with my morning cocktail that consist of two Excedrin Migraine, a 0.5 mg Clonazepam and a bottle of water. I lay there still on my back, concentrating on relaxing; until it takes affect and the pain begins to subside. I won't lie. There have been days when the pain and spasms are so severe that I have thought, "Will today be my last day here?" I don't consider myself a suicidal person, but to be totally truthful I am ashamed to say that, during my darkest times, I have had those thoughts. It's not because my condition is terminal because it's not. What it is, however, is just simply unbearable the majority of the time. Unbearable and, for the most part, misunderstood. With this condition, you quickly learn to internalize in order to appear as normal as possible even though, in your own little world of reality, it's anything but normal. I have come a long way, though. To be truthful, if not for my children, I'm not too sure I would be here today. My husband, well I've always felt he deserved better than to have to walk this journey with me. However, because of them all, I've had the strength to move on and to learn to view things in a different light. So, each day, I gather my strength, adjust my attitude, kick myself out of bed and do it all over again.

This whole nightmare started when I was 49-years-old. I had received Botox three weeks prior for migraines. This was not the first, but the third time, I had received Botox. Everything in my life was finally coming together. We had survived the caregiving challenges and death of my mother-in-law who suffered from lung cancer. Our son had just finished his freshman year in college and received a transfer into his dream college for his sophomore year. Our daughter had graduated with her Ph.D. and was working on her post-doc at one of the top hospitals in the country. She had also started dating an amazing guy, so life was great! Finally, my husband and I were able to start "our lives" together. We had married young and worked so hard, our entire marriage, to get to this point. Then it all went to hell. I had taken the Botox shots in early July of 2014. Approximately three weeks later, I noticed both eyes becoming very heavy and wanting to close, especially when typing on the computer or when watching TV (it's a good thing that I learned to type correctly when I was younger, as I am typing this story now with both eyes closed). The left eye seemed to be worse than the right. I also noticed that the left eye had started twitching. I contacted my eye doctor and she immediately referred me to a Cornea specialist in her group. My biggest fear was that I had Benign Essential Blepharospasms (BEB). He did diagnose me with dry eye and secondary blepharospasms (later it was confirmed by a Neuro Ophthalmologist that I did not have BEB). He treated me for about three months until the spasms began to move down the left side of my face. This caused numbness in my upper left gum and severe sinus pain on both sides. While I was being treated for the eye spasms, I made it a mission to find a Neurologist who would see me. Well, getting into a major hospital in NC to see a Neurologist is impossible without a doctor's referral; the whole process literally takes several months. I looked online and was able to get an appointment immediately with a Neurologist at our local county hospital. Now, I know why. He sucked! I don't think I've ever met a more incompetent and uncaring doctor in my life. He came in, looked at me, performed a few minor touch tests and was done. He never suggested a MRI or anything else. It was "Here's some Xanax and I'll see you in three months." I asked, "Well, do you know what is causing this?" "No." he responded. "Well, could it be menopause?" I asked. His reply was "I don't know. I've seen menopause do some strange stuff. I'll see you in three months." I left there feeling more confused and frustrated than ever. I actually cried all the way home and immediately cancelled that next appointment because I was done with him. Meanwhile, since the spasms continued to move down the left side of my face, the Cornea specialist handed me over to another Ophthalmologist who specialized in Hemifacial Spasms and Blepharospasms treatment. Before leaving his care, I will never forget what he said to me "Sometimes we get older and stuff happens. You just have to learn to deal with it." "What?!" I thought, "So, I'm supposed to accept the fact that I'm losing my independence and having these spasms in my face with my eyes closing up and just move on?" His statement infuriated me. Still, I left without saying anything. By this time, my face would spasm and my eyes would close anytime I looked at something bright like my cell phone, TV, lights, sun, etc. I also could initiate the spasms by touching the upper part of my left lip and, later, any part of the left side of my face. My mouth was becoming involved in the spasms as well, which was even more embarrassing. At least with the eyes, you can somewhat hide behind sunglasses. When I eventually met with the Hemifacial Spasm Ophthalmologist, she was great! She was very much an advocate for me and said that she had never seen anything like my case. She felt there had to be a reason why this was happening. She made me an appointment with an ENT that she knew personally who was with a major hospital with a stellar reputation. Meanwhile, I had made an appointment with my family doctor as well. When I met with my GP, he took one look at me and decided to order a MRI at our local county hospital.

Now, by this time we are well into the fall of 2014. My driving had become extremely limited because my left eye would often close, followed by my right eye. This caused me functional blindness. Simple daily tasks now became super hard chores. Things like cleaning, walking to the mailbox, cooking, shopping, paying bills and putting on makeup were no longer quick and easy tasks. Also, I could forget about watching a movie or television. If I "watched", I really mainly listened. This is when I started to lose so much of my independence. I had always been super independent, a person everyone else depended on. Now, I had to depend on others to take me to appointments. I would still push through daily chores, but by the time my husband would get home from work, I was exhausted. I wanted nothing more than to close my eyes and sleep. Everything had become so difficult that it literally drained me both physically and mentally. Our social life suffered as well. We had always been very social people. I had no desire to spend any time with anyone who was not a close friend of mine. We have a second home on a lake in Virginia, where we loved to entertain. Now that was a chore as well. Even drinking wine, which I always enjoyed, suddenly started to activate the spasms. So, for the most part, I stopped drinking except occasionally. Attending college football games used to be a favorite activity of mine, but it was now something that I could no longer do because it was difficult to walk to the stadium. Even worse was how self-conscious I was about my new spastic appearance. My life had turned into a box that I was trapped in. I just wanted out!

Before I saw the ENT, my first MRI was scheduled. This MRI was somewhat of an experience. Because my husband had taken so much time off work with me, my dad (who lived about fifty minutes away) agreed to bring my mom and take me for my first MRI. Now, let me just add that my mom had been diagnosed with Dementia; however, she was still "with us" mentally at that time.

When we arrived at the county hospital to have the first MRI, the techs were in total confusion as to what I needed done. New at this, I tried to explain that I needed the MRI on my cranial nerves, especially the seventh. Finally, after going back and forth I guess they got it figured out. It was at that point I quickly realized you must be your own advocate. I had the MRI and returned to my doctor's office a few days later for the results. He said, "Your MRI is normal so we now know that you don't have a brain tumor. So, we can all go back to living our normal lives." I literally wanted to scream at him at this point. Don't get me wrong, I've always liked my GP (who has since retired); however, I felt his response to my results were uncaring and just plain dismissive. I thought to myself "What? Go back to our normal lives? Really?! Well maybe YOU can, but I can't! How is that normal?!" Instead, I said nothing again and went on my way. By now, it's been almost five months since my Botox. I felt things had started to improve some. I ended up going to see an endodontist because of the facial pain and found that a root canal that I had ten years prior had not been completed. A root had been missed on an upper left molar and was infected. Could this be my issue? He performed the root canal on the remaining root that was left and I immediately saw some improvement in my upper lip. I could no longer touch it and produce a spasm; however, I still could not touch the left side of my face without a spasm and my eyes closing shut. The numbness in my left upper gum continued as well.

It's now December 2014. I finally had a couple of appointments with the ENT that my new eye doctor set me up with. During both appointments he scoped my sinuses, which was pretty painful. Because of allergies, I could not have the numbing medication that they use. He also ordered a CT scan of my sinuses and, long story short, found nothing wrong. He told me to continue with my Botox. With his recommendation, I returned to the doctor in December of

2014 to receive another round of Botox, now for the Blepharospasms. During this entire time, I constantly asked the doctors "Could it be the Botox?" as all drugs have side effects. They all assured me that my condition had nothing to do with Botox so I continued to use it.

I also want to point out that I visited a neuro physiologist, oral surgeons and a dentist during this time. None of these professionals had ever seen anything like what was happening to me. One oral surgeon believed that, with it starting right after Botox, that maybe Botox could be the problem. Maybe I had a reaction to it. Up to this point, he was the only doctor who suggested that. As most of us with this condition do, I began to Google Hemifacial Spasms and I searched for information on what treatments were available. Once I realized there was a permanent cure called Microvascular Decompression Surgery (MVD), I found a MVD Neurosurgeon at one of the top hospitals on the East Coast. I contacted his office. To my surprise, his nurse called me back after reviewing my written requests and agreed to see me.

By now, it was January of 2015. I was finally in the room with one of the top Neurosurgeons at one of the top hospitals on the East Coast. He examined me and said my Hemifacial Spasm was not like a normal spasm. The most confusing part to him was the fact that my right eye would close shortly after my left eye. There were only spasms on the left side, but, because my right eye was involved, he just was not sure if I had a true Hemifacial Spasm. He ordered a Fiesta MRI, along with hearing tests and an EMG test. He felt like he needed to have more data, which I appreciated. The MRI and hearing tests were performed fairly quickly. The EMG was a different story. I was months away from getting an EMG appointment so I called twice a week to see if anyone had cancelled. Luckily, the staff was super nice about this and even encouraged me to do so. I got lucky. On February 6, 2015 they finally had an opening so my husband took me to the hospital for the EMG. This was one of the hardest days of this entire experience and, still to this day, I find it difficult to talk about.

On the afternoon of February 6, 2015 I arrived at the hospital for the much anticipated EMG. I'm the type of person who tries to make the best out of a situation, especially using humor. It seems to get me through. The MRI and hearing test had already came back normal so everything was banking on this EMG test, which was supposed to be, to my understanding, a sure way to identify a Hemifacial Spasm. They called me back to perform the procedure, while my husband waited in the waiting room. The female doctor came in along with an intern. He stated he was excited to see this because he had heard my case was a very unusual one. I jokingly replied "Well, grab some popcorn and get ready for the freak show." He kind of laughed. For the next forty-five minutes, I laid there while the doctor shocked my face in different areas. Yes, it was somewhat painful, but then came the needles. She stuck them in places in my face and moved them around as her little machine took its readings. I'm talking about super sensitive areas, like under my eye, above my eyebrow, the sides of my face and in my upper lip. All of this was performed on the left side. She didn't say much and then left the room. Soon she reappeared with another doctor who she stated was her boss. The original doctor was confused at my situation. From the way I understood it, with an EMG that detects a Hemifacial Spasm, your face is supposed to react immediately. Mine, reacted right after. It had a delayed reaction and would just go crazy. The second doctor (the boss) decided to not only perform the entire tests again on my left side but on my right side, too. So, I laid there for another forty-five plus minutes of shocking and needles in both sides of my face. Once again, the left side went crazy with delayed reaction and the right side had no reaction what so ever. This second doctor asked if I had suffered any trauma to my face and I replied "no". The pain was intense and I fought back the tears. I had been on that table for almost two hours. I just wanted out of there! Finally, the second doctor and the intern left the room and the original doctor cleaned up my face. I asked her "So, does it look like a Hemifacial Spasm to you?" She replied "Not really. I think it's looking more like Dystonia." Well, not only had I researched Hemifacial Spasm but I had researched Dystonia as well and that word scared me to death. I knew that a lot of the time (from what I read) Dystonia could spread to other parts of your body. Some of the videos I had seen were horrifying and now she's telling me that it looks like I have that! It took every ounce that I had in me not to break down. She continued making small talk, including asking about the weekend and if I had any big plans. I felt like I was in another world. Everything she said had a muffled sound to my brain and honestly I don't even remember what I said to her. Between the physical trauma of the testing and being told I probably had Dystonia, I hit rock bottom that day. I walked out to the waiting room where my husband sat. He said "Are you ready?" I never spoke. "That took a long time", he said. I nodded and dropped my head. He knew not to say anything else. I could no longer hold my emotions inside. Tears were streaming down my face, as that was the longest walk out of the hospital to the parking garage. I felt like I'd just been given a death sentence. By the time we reached the car, I was extremely upset. We sat there, in that parking garage, while I did my best to explain it all to my husband. Neither of us said much on the way home.

One thing about this particular hospital was that they have an online "My Chart" system where you can physically see your test results. I also learned to always request a CD copy of my completed MRI before leaving any office. I noticed that my MRI and hearing tests results came through the "My Chart" system but the EMG never did. I went to the hospital's website and did some research and found out how to manually request the test results. Using the proper forms, it took two times to request the results, but I finally got them. When I eventually received the report, the conclusion, in short form, read "There were no evidence to support Hemifacial Spasm nor were there any evidence to support Dystonia." What??? Thank heavens I ordered this test result because immediately I felt some relief and a little bit of hope. Within three weeks, I was back in to meet with the Neurosurgeon to discuss my results and treatment plan. As I figured from already seeing my results online, he stated that he did not feel comfortable performing MVD surgery on me with the ordered tests indicating it was not a Hemifacial Spasm. The staff was also a little concerned that the EMG could have been compromised by the Botox I had received six weeks prior to the test. The Neurosurgeon referred me to their Movement Disorder Clinic for further evaluation. Once again, it would take six months to get in. This was upsetting to me, as I had been through so much, and I told them that I couldn't wait six months. The surgeon's nurse was awesome and called the doctor's office herself and had me in within four weeks. By the time I started with my Neurologist at the Movement Disorder Clinic, I was another year older. It was March of 2015.

While all of this is happening, my life continued to move forward. That's something this condition, or really any illness doesn't stop for, life. In fact, things in life like stress, anxiety and simply being tired seemed to increase the intensity of my symptoms. The Neurologist tried me on anti-seizure drugs which did not seem to work and made me feel awful. He ended up putting me on 0.5mg of Clonazepam three times a day. I rarely took more than 2 to 2 ½ a day because I would get so tired.

I continued to avoid most social events as much as possible, except those that involved our children. I honestly tried to keep going as much as I could for them, including traveling with them. Wonderful things were happening in both our children's lives and I did not want to miss any of it. I think my biggest fear was being an embarrassment to them, but neither ever made me feel that way. It's sad when you think about having to struggle to get through so many amazing experiences in life. Some you wait forever for. Most importantly, though, I have the memories and that's what matters most to me. Somehow you forget about the struggles when you think back on the memories. They make me smile.

Yes, my personal life continued on with this demon on my back. Our son had started a music career as a singer/songwriter during his college years and was picked up by a Nashville producer. We traveled back and forth to Nashville several times and to other events where he performed. The trips through the Tennessee Mountains were especially tough for me. For some reason, riding in a car causes my eyes to close up and I often get motion sickness. Once, I was so sick that he had to pull off the highway. I'll never forget as I was on my knees sick on the side of the road as he stood over me asking if I was okay. Still, I kept going. I even spent my 50th birthday with him in a recording studio in Nashville. Watching my son excited and working with some amazing and well-known musicians was probably one of the coolest experiences I've ever had. Still, I felt compelled to explain to his producer my condition to avoid embarrassment. I always tried to tuck myself away in the back ground as much as possible as well. You learn fast how to sit so that you don't face people, especially at parties or in restaurants. I was always his "side kick" and we were, at times, in places and rooms with famous people. It was truly a once in a lifetime experience and I am so happy that he allowed me to be a part of that journey with him. Sadly, controlling my face during all of this was a major concern so I often took extra meds. Again, I didn't want to be an embarrassment to him in front of all those people.

Our daughter was also doing well. She became engaged and I was able to travel up north, with my husband, to say 'yes to the dress'. We held a three day engagement party at our lake house in Virginia where we had forty people in and out all weekend. Again, there was always that fear of embarrassment so I had extra Botox thinking that would help. Looking back, it only gave me a frozen face. I helped with preparation of her wedding as much as I could. Mostly, I helped with small miscellaneous things, but she always made me feel a part of the planning. Honestly, she handled 95% of everything, with the help of her fiancée. She even ordered my perfect dress before she found her own. Her career as a doctoral level psychologist had taken off. She went from working at a top hospital to a Clinical Director of a private company and, later, a full time Assistant Teaching Professor. I was able to spend time at her home with her up north and we had an amazing ten day trip together for her new teaching job. It was just her, her dog and I. She would drive for hours and hours and of course most of it I couldn't see. We traveled to different places when she had breaks. I loved spending that time with her. We always seem to find some kind of fun in everything that we do and her patience with me is unconditional.

By the spring of 2015 life continued on and so did the doctors' appointments. My dad spent the next year helping tote me around to appointments when my husband could not. My dad tried to help as much as he could, as my son was away at college and my daughter lived and worked up north. Sadly, my mom's disease continued to progress to the point that she no longer knew me.

My father, who lost sixty pounds caring for my mother could no longer worry about me. Nor, did I expect him to. All of these transitions with my parents made it even more emotionally difficult. Anyone who deals with Dementia or Alzheimer's can fully understand the affect that alone takes on loved ones.

I went on to spend that entire year of 2015 with the Neurologist at the Movement Disorder Clinic. We went back and forth on different things that could possibly be causing my issues. He is an open minded Neurologist, which has been great.

My husband continued to try to balance work and my doctor's appointments and, by the summer, my son was home on break from college. My son spent a lot of time driving me to my doctors' appointments, sitting for hours in his truck. I had MRIs of the brain more than once and even of the neck and spine. Doctors often talked about all sorts of possibilities, but my condition never really fit into one box. Finally, after a year with the Neurologist at the Movement Disorder Clinic, he contacted the Chief of Neurosurgery. My Neurologist at the Movement Disorder Clinic sent me back to him. He told Neurosurgeon that he really felt it was a Hemifacial Spasm.

After that yearlong evaluation at the Movement Disorder Clinic and different MRIs/MRAs, the Neurosurgeon finally decided he would try the MVD surgery. Because they could not find any compression on the MRI (later I was told a lot don't show up) he was up front with me that my condition was very abnormal and he could not promise that he could help me. He would do his best to try. That was all that I could ask for.

It was February of 2016 and they set the surgery date for March 24, 2016. This was six weeks before our only daughter was to be married. I was really worried about this because missing that event would have killed me. They assured me I'd be fine in six weeks to attend so I signed up for it. Prior to the surgery, I attended her bridal shower and tried to stay in the back of the room away from people as much as possible. See, most people still didn't know what was going on with me, but they had started to notice the withdrawn personality I was exhibiting.

The MVD Surgery:
I was admitted to the hospital on a Wednesday, the day prior to the procedure. I have to admit that I felt very confident in the hospital's preparation of the surgery. I had already been through all of my pre-op a couple of weeks prior. My hospital room was private and even had sleeping quarters for my husband. We settled in late that afternoon and an entire staff from nurses, surgical residents to the anesthesiologist came in as a group and explained my procedure in great detail to me. They even went over the risks and discussed exactly what actions would be performed if any problems did occur. After they left, the nurse had me shower and wash my hair and body in an antibacterial solution to prepare me for surgery at 6:00 a.m. the next morning. Once settled into bed that night, a nurse came in, prepared my numerous IVs and administered the first dose of a certain type of steroid. I don't recall what it was; however, it was not like anything I had ever had before. The nurse prepared me for the very weird and uncomfortable feelings I would have in certain areas of my body. She did not lie! It was like I was literally being eaten up by fire ants. Luckily, it did not last longer than ten or fifteen minutes, but this happened again with every dose. My husband settled into his quarters watching television as I laid in the bed waiting for the next day. I can't really say what I was feeling. By this point, I

think I had just become numb, but that night I experienced an unexpected spiritual occurrence. It was one of the most comforting things that had ever happened to me. After that experience, I had no anxiety or fear of going through with the surgery. I knew everything would go fine.

The day of the surgery, Thursday, they came and took me down at around 5:30 a.m. My husband and I met with the surgeon prior to going in. He explained that he was doing another MVD in the operating room beside me, but assured me that he would be the one doing the actual surgery. Yes, I asked! Being a large teaching hospital, I'm sure a resident performed some of the other tasks. The first twenty four hours after the surgery are pretty much a blur, as I was in ICU. I don't do well with anesthesia and they knew that going in. They tried to mix a proper "cocktail" as they called it to keep me from getting so sick; however, it did not work. I was vomiting a lot for the first twenty four hours. Of course, with stitches in your brain, that's not the best thing. I also had what we jokingly called a "brain drain" inserted in the spinal area to drain any excess fluid off. My son came to visit me on that Friday. My daughter and her then fiancée drove in from up north on that Saturday. Neither of my children does well with graphic "medical" stuff so the "brain drain" was not a favorite! In regards to my spasms, I did not wake up spasm free. The surgeon explained that he found a main vessel that was running parallel to the CN VII and was actually touching it. He did not see any actual nerve damage, but explained that there could be some, as nerves are like fiber optic cables and they can't always see the damage. He inserted two Teflon pads to separate the vessel and the CN VII. After the surgery, I could touch my face without stimulating a spasm so that was about a fifty percent improvement. My eyes, though, were still not working correctly. After days of steroids, insulin shots (because of the steroids), shots in my stomach for blood clot prevention and pain meds the "brain drain" was removed and I was released from the hospital. That was Easter Sunday evening 2016.

I felt like my recovery at home went quiet well. My husband stayed home with me for the first week and took care of me. It was a lot easier than I had expected. I just had to be very careful for the first six weeks. Neighbors and friends brought food, which was very nice. Even though, I would tire easily I was able to fully participate and attend our daughter's festivities and wedding which was five hours away six weeks later. I was still having problems with my eyes closing up, but I was able to once again hide behind my sunglasses because it was an outdoor ceremony. All in all, it was a beautiful occasion and I'm so thankful for every single minute of it! Most importantly to me, she was able to have her perfect wedding.

After that first surgery and still not spasm free, I spent the next two and half years searching for answers. I continued to still be under the care of my Neurologist at the Movement Disorder Clinic. Since the spasms never truly went away, I returned back to the Neurosurgeon who ordered another MRI. Once again it was clear and he said he felt that it was too dangerous to go back in. He sent me through a Bio-Feedback program for months, which I had no success with. I started seeing a chiropractor as well. She helped relieve a little stress from the tight muscles in the neck from the spasms, but the services soon became too costly. I also saw a well-known TMJ specialist in NC. She ran a CT scan that indicated that I had TMJ with the left jaw bone pushed up against my ear. She ordered a CT scan to see if it was pushing on a cranial nerve outside the brain. She even built me a mouthpiece to attempt to adjust my jaw to see if that would help. She had no success with either.

I also traveled up north, with my husband, to another top MVD Neurosurgeon in the US for a second opinion. His MRI was intense! I have to say, I've never felt anything like that before. Prior to seeing him, he had me scheduled for an EMG. When the EMG fired late, like it had before, I knew it was not going to be what I had hoped for. In fact, the doctor performing the EMG commented on how weird it was that my face had such a delayed reaction. It's sad when you're hoping to see something wrong on your brain MRI. Once it was time to meet with the Neurosurgeon, it was just as I suspected it would be. He showed my husband and me the MRI. He even showed us the Teflon pads on the scan that were placed during my MVD surgery. He said he was one hundred percent certain that there were no compressions inside the brain. Like my previous Neurosurgeon, he said it was just too dangerous to go back in. I told him that every doctor I had seen said that they had never seen anyone quite like me before. He stated he had seen a few, but only a few. I really can't say I left disappointed; not getting answers had been the norm for me for years.

When you go through something like this desperation often sets in. You will try anything or any type of doctor to figure it out. I've seen every type of professional from Spine doctors, Chiropractors, Oral Surgeons, Dentists, TMJ specialists, ENTs, Rheumatologists, several various Eye doctors, Psychologists and yes, many Neuro doctors and Surgeons as well. All in all, I've seen 60 doctors and have medical bills over $450,000 to this date. Yes, I have health insurance, but there have still been large sums of money due in deductibles and not everything has been covered. I know my health puts a lot of pressure on my husband, as his job and health care benefits are now crucial to us.

So where am I today? I am still searching, praying and hoping that one day I can see the light at the end of my tunnel. I work to control the spams (and usually pain) all day long. My eyes, closing up, are still my biggest battle, but I continue to get through each day by doing my daily tasks. Yes, I might be a lot slower than I used to be, but I get it done. I'm still on Clonazepam daily and am constantly trying to reduce my intake levels, but it's tough. I've tried CBD oil with 4% THC, while visiting California and it actually works well, but is short lived. Sadly, it's not legal in North Carolina. I was also recently tested for Sjogren's Disease via a biopsy and it came back positive but at a level one. My Rheumatologist ran about twelve other blood tests in order to be able to properly diagnose me with Sjogren's Disease, but they all came back either at a low level or negative. He's asked that I discontinue the Botox since it seems to no longer be working. In fact, at times I get worse when using it. Plus, there's still that lingering fact that I was totally normal until three weeks after Botox injections via a head/neck specialist for migraines. So, I'm now discontinuing the Botox treatments. Still, I try to have hope. My Neurologist has recently referred me to his colleague, a Pain Specialist Neurologist who works with facial pain, especially CN V, for an additional evaluation and pain treatment. May I also add that he is a scientist as well. The Neurologists have all said from the beginning, because of the gum numbness/sensory/pain issues that CN V is involved along with CN VII. With a nine month waiting list to see this Pain Specialist Neurologist, I was very fortunate that my Neurologist got me in with him within weeks. I have to say, as of now, I've been impressed. He very much is "thinking outside the box" in regards to my condition and this is something that I desperately need. While I have a team of doctors now, he is the leader of my treatment plan which includes consulting with other specialists. We are in the process of trying several different medications and treatment options, one being multiple days at a time of Steroid IV infusions.

All in all, this is by far, the worst and hardest battle that I've ever had to fight in my life. I guess that's because I've never really been able to see the "light" at the end of the tunnel that I've been so desperately seeking. I'm constantly praying that one day that will change. I have, though, learned so much through this experience. I've learned who my true friends are. While you may have many friends, you will have very few "ride or die" friends who stick with you. Those are the friends who really try to understand what is happening to you. They are your biggest cheerleaders. They are constantly there for you. Those are the friends who do not pity you, but are the ones who say "you amaze me!" Those are the friends you can laugh with about your condition, as it doesn't freak them out. I'm so thankful for those very few friends. I've also learned that my husband really took our marriage vows serious as he has stood beside me through this entire journey. He has lost time from work, it's upset his entire world and there have been times when I've been so miserable and broken that I've run him away. Still, he came back. It's funny because I used to joke around saying I wish God would give me a Plastic Surgeon as a child or in-law. Instead, God gave me a Psychologist. He gave me my daughter. I guess he knew something that I didn't. She's been there to guide me and teach me so much about handling this condition. I'm sharing this in hopes that maybe it will help others as well. She's taught me that I have to slow down and "put my airplane mask on first" before I can worry or help anyone else. I need to take care of myself first. This has been difficult for me, but I'm getting there. She's taught me that, while never giving up hope, I must also have acceptance. I've learned to stop living in the past and dwelling on what I had because I may never have it again. Instead, I am alive and, as long as I'm alive, I have a future. So, I need to plan that future. As hard as it's been I've even made some big travel trips. I've had my son's support and patience. He's been there for me through so many appointments. I'll never forget the day a test result came back negative once again. I had so much hope and was upset. I'll always remember his words to me, "So what are WE going to do next?" Not YOU, but WE. Hearing that one sentence gave me so much comfort. I don't know if my son will ever realize the extent of the peace that the sound of his music brings to me or how I depend on it to help me drive my car. It's like I'm not alone. He is with me.

In a sense, I've been very lucky. I've had an amazing support system. I can't express enough how important that is for someone going through this life changing (and often debilitating) condition. I've had some great doctors who have truly tried to help me. However, as a mother, it always comes back to my children regarding why I've kept going and who I am today. I credit my daughter for saving my mind with her guidance and my son for saving my soul with his music.

Trixie

My name is Trixie. I'm a 42 year old female from Manila, Philippines, and this is my Hemifacial Spasm story.

My Hemifacial Spasms started 11 years ago, when I was a graduating medical student, rotating as a medical intern in a busy hospital in Manila, Philippines. I was sleeping an average of four hours a night because of medical studies, and medical rotations kept us interns up for 36 hours every three days. As a medical student, I tried to keep a balance between studies and health so I played badminton weekly with my friends. At one time, I was playing with an acquaintance who was playing very competitively. He accidentally hit the back of my head with his badminton racket after going after the shuttle cock. It was a very strong hit and I found myself down on the floor for several minutes.

Months later, after that hit, my lower right eyelid started twitching uncontrollably. I sought a consultation from a local neurologist who told me not to mind the twitching since it was due to sleepless nights. One day, I was interviewing some patients when a patient exclaimed, "Your illness is worse than mine, you should have yourself checked." I didn't realize that my spasms had already gotten that bad until that moment. I had myself checked by neurologists, and they were not sure of what I had. I went through numerous MRI's, EMG-NCVs, which all came out with normal results. One neurologist concluded that I had high levels of anxiety and prescribed me haloperidol, a drug which is usually prescribed for schizophrenia. I refused to believe that what I had was a psychosomatic disorder. I knew that there was something causing the uncontrollable twitching, but the neurologists that I consulted couldn't find any reason for the twitching. At that time, I was also in an awful relationship, which caused me a lot of stress and anxiety. This person made me believe that, because of my spasms; no man would love and accept me for what I have. Sleeping became difficult because the spasms were waking me up with the constant nagging. Smiling was difficult because any movement in the mouth triggered my spasms. I dropped out of medical school and ended the awful relationship. I went into depression.

My mother saw what was happening to me, and she was very concerned. She encouraged me to visit my sister who is a family medicine doctor in Pennsylvania. I flew to the United States to give myself a much needed break and seek resolution for my depression. Upon arriving in the US, my sister pricked me up from the airport. When she saw my spasms, she broke down into tears and promised me that we would look for answers for my spasms together. And so, every night, we would surf the internet looking for possible diagnoses and solutions. We then came across an online Hemifacial support group, and we knew we had our diagnosis. We knew coming across this page was a miracle because the Hemifacial Spasm center in Pittsburgh, which was constantly being mentioned, was only one hour away from my sister's town. Immediately, we knew we had to book an appointment.

Two weeks later, I found myself face to face with a neurosurgeon from the prestigious hospital in Pittsburgh, and after a MRI and EMG NCV, he confirmed the Hemifacial Spasm diagnosis. The neurosurgeon told me that I needed MVD surgery, which was the only permanent solution for my spasms. I didn't know what to do because I didn't have insurance coverage in the United States so everything would have to be paid out-of-pocket. Since I was a student, I didn't have that amount of money, even with the 3rd world country discount given by U.S. hospitals. Again, I went into depression.

My parents, who were in the Philippines at that time, assured me that they would help me get the operation. And by God's grace and mercy, they were able to come up with the money needed for my operation. On January 17, 2009, I had my MVD surgery. I was immediately spasm free and it gave me back my life.

Two months later, I was back in medical school to finish my medical studies. I had the renewed energy and assurance of a new life, and I aimed at becoming a neurologist who would treat Hemifacial Spasms. I labored day and night, studying to be a doctor, when to my horror and surprise, my spasms returned six months later. I immediately stopped school and decided to put my medical dream on the shelf permanently. I took it to myself to sleep 8 hours a day, take an afternoon nap, take vitamin b complex and exercise daily. My spasms decreased to a minimal level, although it did not recede completely. I shifted careers to real estate, and decided to focus on my health. At this time, I rekindled a friendship with a man whom I knew from my teenage years. He is a wonderful, thoughtful, simple, God fearing and handsome man who didn't mind my spasms. He is a man who looked beyond my spasms and appreciated me for myself. A year later, we got married and I prayed to God to have a spasm-free wedding day. God is good, and he granted my wish. Amidst my fears of twitching and spasming at all my guests, I walked down the aisle with a big smile on my face, and no spasms!

For a few months, I remained spasm free until I had my first pregnancy. The spasms started progressing and even surpassed the level of before my MVD surgery. My neurologist in the Philippines told me that it was possible that the pregnancy hormones were triggering my spasms. I was elated that I was having a baby, but at the back of my mind, I had my fears about my spasms. My husband wanted to take lots of photos to document the pregnancy, but even though I wanted to take lots of photos, each photo brought anxiety because of the spasms. I still could not accept the fact that my spasms were back, and they were back with a vengeance.

I gave birth to my beautiful baby girl. I started accepting the fact that my spasms were back and they were at a level worse than before until I started having unbearable headaches. I went through so many things suggested to me: Zen meditation, acupuncture, yoga, taichi, Botox injections, functional medicine, but nothing gave a permanent solution. At this time, I became a member of the Hemifacial Spasms International and Worldwide groups. I started reading about a famous surgeon in Pennsylvania with a very high success rate. With my headache starting to get unbearable, my mother and my husband suggested that I visit him. Two months later, I found myself in front of the famous doctor, in the same Hemifacial Spasm center as my previous

MVD surgery, in the renowned hospital in Pittsburgh. He looked at my MRI scans and told me that there was still a compression in my brain, and that he needed to do another MVD surgery. I went back to the Philippines not hoping for anything because again, we would have to pay out of pocket for this second MVD surgery. I decided to just bear the pain. I received Botox treatments to ease the pain, as we couldn't afford another surgery, especially since my husband and I have the financial responsibility towards our growing family. But God works in mysterious ways. My parents informed me that they would pay for my surgery again since they couldn't bear seeing their youngest child in pain and suffering from spasms. I was amazed at how much love they had to give. My father-in-law also offered to share in the expenses, and that's when I realized the goodness and love of the people around me. Six months later, I found myself under the knife for my second MVD surgery, being operated on by the famous doctor.

One year later, I am still not spasm free, but I found my spasms greatly reduced. At least the headache was relieved and I realized that maybe the good Lord had a purpose for keeping my spasms in my face. I started the Hemifacial Spasms Organization Philippines, a Hemifacial Spasms group for Filipinos and Philippine Residents. I found it amazing that there are so many Filipinos who have this condition, and everybody had the same story. We were all lonely, depressed, and we all found refuge and solace in each other. Many of our members could not afford treatment for Hemifacial Spasms, Botox or medical treatment, especially since the minimum pay per day in the Philippines is about 10 U.S. dollars. Therefore, a lot of our members would just tolerate the condition, depression and prejudice by others, and pray that it goes away. On August 19th, 2018, together with one of the biggest hospitals in Makati, Philippines, we had our first Hemifacial Spasms summit in the Philippines. We gave free Botox treatment to all the Hemifacial Spasm participants. It was also the first time that we had more than 50 Hemifacial Spasm patients in the same room, feeling at home and without fear of being judged by others. Currently, we have 319 members and our group is still growing!

Two years after my MVD surgery, I have stopped complaining about the spasms. Yes, they are still there, and occasionally I still get headaches, but I know now that there is a reason why I continue to have them despite my two MVD surgeries. I have a mission in the Philippines to help my fellow Hemifacial Spasm sufferers. Yes, I do get spasms when I talk to others but I don't feel embarrassed anymore. I just laugh at my spasms now. I've learned to embrace and accept this.

Susan Nofi

My name is Susan Nofi. I'm a 73-year-old female from Massachusetts, USA and this is my Hemifacial Spasm story.

It started in 1982. My eyelid on the left side of my face started twitching and little by little the twitching started moving down the left side of my face. This happened to me pre-internet days, where perhaps I could have looked it up if it were now. I made appointments with doctors to get an idea of what was causing this. I had many tests and was put on some medications, including a muscle relaxant, which affected me in a very bad way. Having small children, the feelings that I experienced were not good. The doctors were clueless as to what was causing this. Finally, the doctors thought that perhaps all of this was in my mind. They suggested that I see a psychiatrist, who might be able to help me. After seeing him for a while, I just couldn't afford to go anymore.

One day, my friend mentioned that a friend of hers was having a hard time going to work and being among his co-workers due to facial spasms. He found a doctor in a well-known hospital, who operated on him and the spasms stopped. My husband and I decided to see this particular Neurologist and then we made the decision that I would go through with the MVD surgery. The surgeon that I had hoped to see was quite far away. Being that our children were still young, we opted to go with another Neurosurgeon. If I had known then what I know now, I would have never let him do my first MVD surgery on September 8th, 1983.

It turns out that I was only the second patient that this Neurosurgeon had performed a MVD surgery on! I came out paralyzed on my left side and my heart was acting up. My spasms were still with me and I ended up in the hospital for three weeks. I couldn't walk and had physical therapy for quite a while. I still have weakness on my left side, which affects my balance. One good thing did come out of this awful time in my life, though. We ended up seeing a doctor in Pittsburgh, who was a specialist in the Hemifacial Spasm field. We gave it a lot of thought before making the decision to see him.

MVD surgery number two! We met with the neurosurgeon that would be doing my second MVD surgery and walked away very impressed by his knowledge in the Hemifacial Spasm field. I wrote a letter to the doctor's office regarding his credentials and he told me the success rate with this operation was greater than 95% with some other minor risks. After giving it considerable thought, I contacted his office and my MVD surgery was scheduled for March 24th, 1985. The staff was very nice and accommodating.

Well, the day finally arrived and I went through all the steps of admission. The surgeon was doing four MVD's surgeries that day and I was to be his second. The staff, in the operating room, was wonderful and the surgeon did talk to me prior to the surgery. He was a wonderful human being. The next thing that I knew, I was in the recovery room. They didn't keep me there for long as I was feeling very well. I was taken to my room and not only was I feeling well, my face was CALM. I had done so well that my surgeon took me to see a couple of other patients who were having their MVD surgeries as well. For all that had gone wrong with the first

MVD surgery, everything went incredibly well with the second one. I credit that to having a Neurosurgeon who had experience in this field.

Back then, the hospital stay was longer than it is now. My husband went back home as he had to go back to work and my mom came to keep me company. She was very happy to see me in such good shape. She stayed at a place that was called the "Family House". They provided a room, meals and rides to/from the hospital. We flew back home when I was released and my good life began. I went back to my usual routines, taking care of my family and returning to work.

I was spasm free for ten years, when suddenly, the spasms came back with a vengeance. They were bad around my mouth and got worse when I smiled. It hit me very hard and I went back to that place emotionally where I was before. I was hiding from others at times and feeling very down. I put up with the spasms for a few years. They acted up during the night and I felt like hitting my face to make them stop. One day, my daughter called and, while talking to her, I started to cry on the phone. A couple of days later, she did some research on the computer and found the HFSA group. I looked them up and felt such comfort when reading other people's struggles and realizing that I wasn't alone. I made an appointment with the Neurosurgeon that had done my second MVD surgery.

Third MVD surgery! October 3rd, 2002. The surgeon and I talked for quite a while beforehand. He made it very clear that the third MVD surgery would be quite difficult. Apparently he felt that what had been placed by the neurosurgeons prior were perhaps contributory to pushing the nerve into a large vein causing the spasms to start up again. They did quite a bit during my surgery, which was explained by a written surgical report. He said that I tolerated the surgery well and left the operating room in satisfactory condition. While in the recovery room nausea kicked in and got worse as time went on, accompanied with a terrible headache. I pretty much kept my head still throughout the day and my eyes closed, which seemed to help. When they brought my dinner tray, my daughter had to take it out of my room because the smell made me feel even worse. I was told that this is normal and it would pass. Friday night, I threw up the little bit that I had consumed that day.

Second day post-op, Saturday, October 5, 2002. I found myself seemingly feeling a little better. However, I still had a headache and some nausea. Also, I had not had very much of an appetite. I was able to eat a little breakfast and half a sandwich for dinner. Everyone kept telling me how great I looked and how well I was doing. I perked up as the day went on and peeked at myself, which was scary. I did notice that the Hemifacial side had a great deal of weakness and flutters. I was told that this would get better as time went on. I must say my face was very calm, which was a great feeling. I went for a couple of little strolls holding on to my husband and daughter. Because of the weakness on my Hemifacial Spasm side, my eye wasn't closing all the way. I was given a cream to put in it at night and my eye was taped shut.

Third day post-op, Sunday, October 6, 2002. A physician's assistant came in to see me bright and early that morning. I knew he was there for the great unveiling. He pulled the tape off my incision and the tape didn't let go easily. It hurt quite a bit until he got it all off. The incision was about 12" long. I was told that I was being discharged that day. I needed to shower and wash my hair, per the doctor's orders. We left the hospital and went to Hawthorne Suites. We had pizza delivered and it felt so good to enjoy food again.

Fourth day post-op, Monday, October 7, 2002.
I spent the day relaxing and I must admit that I was feeling much better than I thought I would! The following day, we had a follow up appointment with my surgeon. After that, we would begin our journey home.

Fifth day post-op, Tuesday, October 8, 2002.
My surgeon came into the room and we talked about the noticeable weakness on my Hemifacial Spasm side. He felt that it should improve. We also talked about exercises or therapy that I could do after a few weeks. We said our goodbyes and I started the long journey home.

The weakness progressed, which affected my eye in very bad ways. I got to the point that I couldn't tolerate outside lighting, even on cloudy days. I went to see an eye specialist and he felt that gold eyelid weight would help the situation. It did help with outdoor lighting and any kind of bright objects. I also went through a long period of eye infections, which required a doctor's visit. In addition, I visited the ER with a severe eye infection.

After a period of time, my gold weight was removed. The left side of my eye was given a couple of stiches, which left the eye quite a bit smaller and prevented the eye from being over exposed. Little by little, the left side of my face got weaker and weaker. I've done exercises and gone for speech therapy. Unfortunately, neither helped. People have asked if I've had a stroke. It truly bothers me when people take pictures, because my smile is pretty much gone. I feel freakish at times. I have to say; it affects me emotionally quite a bit. The one thing that I will always be grateful for, though, is that I'm spasm free!!!!!

Shirl Boatman
"Hemifacial Spasm is no friend of mine"

My name is Shirl Boatman. I am 59 years old and live in Lenox, IL, USA. This is my Hemifacial Spasm story.

Have you ever had that unexplained, infrequent flutter or twitch of the eyelid that lasted 1-2 minutes before ending just as quickly as it started? In July 2010, that twitch in my right eye started me down a path that I never anticipated. I never considered myself model material, but I had great self confidence that I was "pretty". Little did I know how much that self-image would change over the course of the next nine years. The eyelid flutter became more frequent even though at first it only lasted 1- 2 minutes each time and was still somewhat unnoticeable by others.

Over the next 18 months or so, the flutter began to last longer and longer. Before I knew it, that involuntary movement of my right eyelid had migrated to areas to the right of and just below my right eye. It quickly became annoying. I couldn't imagine what was going on. With each passing day, I was looking for answers and the only explanation I could conceive was eye strain. The largest majority of my adult life had been spent in front of a computer. Perhaps decades of this continual exposure to a computer monitor was having an impact.

Fast forward to 2012 and it was time for my annual physical exam with my primary care physician. During this exam, I mentioned my issue to him. It had progressed to the point that it was now visible to others. He didn't know what it was, but told me I "wouldn't die from it"! Great bedside manner!

Shortly thereafter, I went to my optometrist and asked him about it. Believe it or not, he basically had the same answer as my primary physician, "I don't know what it is, but you won't die from it." This was frustrating, as both of the medical professionals I had consulted with didn't have a clue what was going on and didn't understand the "mental" strain it was having on me.

As a result of the lack of medical knowledge on my condition, the next course of action could only be to "Google" my symptoms. By now I had noticed the area affected had begun to increase. It was moving horizontally to my hairline and downward on my cheek. After many hours of searching and searching, I was not having any success. The best I was able to find: *"Researchers have speculated on several causes – including misdirected brain activity, tired eyes, too much caffeine, certain drug withdrawals, stress, irritation or dry eyes. However, the cause of most eyelid twitches remains unknown."*

I didn't give up and kept searching until; finally, one day there it was…Hemifacial Spasm (HFS). I experienced so many of the symptoms described. Now I was armed with a possible name and could search with more intelligence. I found numerous postings by individuals who were discussing their experiences with HFS. This was not a true diagnosis, just my own diagnosis based on my hours of online research.

By August 2013, it had progressed to the point that it was now sometimes obvious in photos.

At my physical exam in 2014, I insisted to my physician (a different physician than before), that I needed to see a specialist and asked if could he recommend a Neurologist. He finally referred me to a Neurologist and I made my appointment. She immediately diagnosed Hemifacial Spasm (HFS) and recommended Botox. I broke down and cried because, at long last, I had a medical diagnosis (which, by the way, confirmed my diagnosis).

We began the long process of getting approval from the insurance company for Botox injections. After a couple of months, my insurance company approved the treatment and I began my first injections of Botox on August 4th, 2014. The Neurologist explained that it could take 1-2 weeks to show any signs of improvement and effects would only last up to three months. She injected Botox just above my brow line, on my eyelid, to the right of my eye, just below the eye and on my upper cheek. She minimally injected the left side as well to "balance" the effects. Well, about two weeks after the injection, I started noticing that my right eye was very dry during my waking hours. I wondered if I was blinking often enough. Looking in the mirror, I attempted to see if I was blinking; however, this proved impossible. When my husband returned from work that evening, I asked him to watch me and see if I was blinking. Sure enough that right eye was never blinking. While the Botox stopped the twitching, it also stopped the natural blinking, thus causing a dry eye. As time progressed, the Botox began to cause my cheek and lip to droop when I attempted to smile. I could only make a half-smile. Then there was the "freezing" effects of Botox on my right side. While my right eye remained open, I no longer had control of my right cheek and right side of my lip.

I continued with Botox injections for about nine months. My last injection was in May 2015, as I decided the side effects of Botox were worse for me than HFS.

My condition became more profound and the smile I once knew was now a fading memory. It was rare for me to allow a photo to be taken of me because the results were less than favorable. The twitching had become so exaggerated that the right side of my face was twitching more often than not. It was waking me up at night. I could "hear" the twitching in my ear. Changing positions in bed, pressing firmly on different areas of my face and head, breathing slowly and rhythmically – none of these measures provided any relief from the twitching.

I could no longer wear makeup because it was nearly impossible to place eye shadow or mascara on my right eye.

By 2016, HFS had engulfed my life and I was in an emotional and psychological battle with myself to remain positive and cheery. I have always been a social person so I refused to allow this "affliction" to turn me into a mushroom, isolating myself from the world. But I certainly did not feel "pretty" any longer and I was continually embarrassed in pubic by my facial expressions. When I would share this with friends and family, they would respond, "Oh gosh, we hardly notice it; we think you are pretty." Well, I realize that, because they love me, they were trying to make me feel better. However, every time I looked in the mirror, it was difficult not to notice. I knew they saw it as well.

In 2017, I was conversing with someone who I had recently met at a social gathering. She looked at me and said, "What is wrong with your eye?" That made me feel really good because she noticed and wasn't afraid to ask about it. I began to explain it to her and I thanked her for being so honest and asking me.

I was recently traveling for work and was with a coworker from another location who I hadn't seen in over a year. He greeted me with, "What is wrong? Do you not feel well?" I said, "I feel fine, why?" He said, "Your eye." Again, I was appreciative that he asked about it. I proceeded to tell him about it and he said, "Oh, I am so sorry to hear that. Is there a cure?" Well, those of us with HFS know the answer to that question…

How is it affecting me today?
- HFS prevents me from going to sleep quickly because of the endless twitching of my eye and cheek and "hearing" the twitching in my ear.
- It wakes me up once I have finally fallen asleep and prevents me from going back to sleep.
- Vertigo has become an issue for me as well. Sometimes just lying in bed will set off the vertigo. There is no rhyme or reason to the vertigo. It will hit me when lying, sitting, standing, etc. But it is random. I am a cyclist and I am growing alarmed that someday I may be unable to safely ride the bike or even drive a car.
- There are times when working is difficult, as I can barely see the computer.
- I also have sleep apnea and wear a CPAP. When the twitching is out of control, it affects the fit of my CPAP mask.

I am becoming more and more interested in Microvascular decompression (MVD), also known as the Jannetta procedure. This is a surgery to relieve abnormal compression of a cranial nerve causing trigeminal neuralgia, glossopharyngeal neuralgia, or Hemifacial Spasm. I am so grateful for the Hemifacial Spasm group on Facebook. This group has educated me in so many ways by allowing me to read about others who have been plagued with this same awful curse. With this group and the sharing of their stories by others, it has made me feel like I am not alone. The information and photos shared by so many have taken me much closer to picking up the phone and calling one of the top MVD Neurosurgeons in the U.S. to start the process of determining if I am a candidate for MVD and, if so, what my next steps will be.

I am often haunted by the words of my medical doctor and optometrist in the early stages trying to get a diagnosis, "I don't know what it is, but you won't die from it." No, not physical death, but I have died a little each day emotionally and psychologically as my HFS continues to advance.

Hopefully, more research will result in a less intrusive "cure" for this disease. While HFS has been by my side for the last nine years and would normally constitute a "friendship", HFS is no friend of mine. I am so ready to kick HFS to the curb, remaining only in my memory. It is my dream that the next chapter of my life will be written without the presence of HFS. At the writing of this article, I am not sure yet what the path will be to get me there.

Sharina Samarista

My name is Sharina Samarista. I'm a 30-year-old female from Camarines Sur, Philippines. This is my Hemifacial Spasm story.

It started with the usual twitching on my right eyelid while I was preparing for my Nurse Licensure Examination following my graduation from college in 2009. I ignored the twitching because I thought it wasn't serious. A year later, the twitching became more obvious and started to cause discomfort in my face. I became more conscious of it and worried. I decided to consult an ophthalmologist because I am also near sighted and have a stigmatism. I was told that the twitching was not connected to my other eye problems so I consulted a general physician. The physician referred me to a neurologist who prescribed Rivotril to alleviate the spasms. I also underwent an MRI and MRA to further evaluate what may be causing the involuntary twitching. The results were normal with one exception. My 7th cranial nerve was compressed by a blood vessel, thus causing the spasms. At this time, I was diagnosed with a right Hemifacial Spasm.

I'm a nurse, but my family and I still needed a detailed explanation of my condition because it is rare. Following the diagnosis, I began Botox injections to ease or calm my face. I received Botox around once or twice a year depending on the longevity of the previous injection. Back then, I was also told by my neurologist that there was a surgical procedure that could fix me. The MVD surgery that he was referring to was too expensive. Due to the cost of the surgery, I endured Botox injections for a long time. We were aware that Botox was not a cure for my condition and that it would require reoccurring sessions because it only paralyzed the affected muscles. The injections were really expensive and each one required travel from our town to Manila (the capital of the Philippines) because Botox was not common in my country. We didn't mind spending money to allow my face to calm down, though.

To be honest, this condition greatly affected me emotionally and socially. I am a very sociable person, but I became withdrawn as my condition worsened. It also affected my profession. There was a time when I decided to make the shift from working in a hospital setting to a more confined work place so that I did not need to interact with other people. I was tired of explaining my condition. Yes, I felt ashamed, but I didn't have a choice. I had to continue living because this had become a part of me.

Then I discovered an international and local Hemifacial Spasm group on Facebook. I began conversing with other members and was glad to see that I was not alone. I also found out that MVD surgeries were being performed in the Philippines so I started contacting patients who had undergone the surgery.

Last year, we found a great neurosurgeon. He had performed many MVDs so I scheduled an appointment with him. I personally wanted (badly) to have the surgery. Finally, after so many years of suffering, I had my MVD surgery on February 27, 2019 in Manila, Philippines.

I did not wake up spasm-free. I was told that this was because I had this condition for almost a decade. My neurosurgeon said that the procedure was successful; however, there are cases like mine where it will take some time for my system to adjust. "Just be patient", he told me. As of now, I am four months post MVD surgery and I can say that I am almost 100% spasm-free. Thank, God! I am really grateful to my Hemifacial Spasm journey (both positive and negative) and to all the people that became a part of it.

Joe Pane

My Name is Joe Pane. I'm a 51-year-old, married father of three from Melbourne, Australia. This is my Hemifacial Spasm story so far.

It all started as a minor twitch in my right-side eye in July 2014. After noticing the spasms, I went to see my local general practitioner (GP) who assured me that there was nothing to worry about. He said it was "maybe caused by stress". The spams continued for a couple more months before progressing to a "pulse sensation" in the right side of my head while I slept. This was quite annoying. I returned to my GP and asked for a referral to a specialist who could have a look at me. I was connected with a Neurologist at a private hospital who ordered an MRI. The MRI was pretty daunting the first time, as I didn't know what type of condition I had. It was this Neurologist who diagnosed me with Hemifacial Spasm. He said that there was nothing that could be done for my condition and prescribed me Epilepsy tablets called Tegretol. I didn't agree with him so I went back to my GP and asked to see another specialist at a different hospital. I wanted to get a second opinion.

Next, I saw a Neurosurgeon at a leading private hospital in Melbourne. He immediately performed another MRI and the results suggested that I had a compressed nerve. These findings confirmed that I had a Hemifacial Spasm. The Neurosurgeon sent me to a Neurologist who prescribed Botox injections. I became especially nervous during this time and started to search my condition on Google. I eventually found this Hemifacial Spasms Facebook Group and discovered that there were a lot of similar people like me. Lucky me, 5 out of 100,000 people have this condition and I was one of them. I began receiving Botox Injections once every three months for the next fifteen months, which was effective. Others would really notice when the Botox would wear off after two and a half months, though.

The thumping in my head while I slept would not go away even with the Botox treatments. Not being able to get a full night's sleep was causing me grief. I then made an appointment to go back and see the Neurosurgeon and we booked a MVD Operation for the 15th of December in 2015. I booked it on this date because I am self-employed and this would be the best time, allowing me to recover over the Christmas Break. It was a scary situation, as I had never been in Hospital in my 47 years alive. The operation went well; I recovered well and was spasm free.

The spasms started to come back around three months post-surgery and got progressively worse. I decided to see a leading Professor of Neuroscience at the same hospital to get yet another opinion. He performed another MRI on me and found that the Teflon pad, placed during the MVD surgery, had actually moved. It was a fine line when they placed the Teflon pad into my skull; too much is bad, but not enough can cause the pad to shift and mine did just that.

I returned to using Botox, which seemed to work well as it had when I previously used it. However, the spasms and my "head thumping" were causing me grief so I decided to have another MVD surgery in December 2016. During the operation, the Professor who performed my operation put a new Teflon Pad in position. Again, I recovered even better than the first time, as I knew what to expect the second time around. As I recovered, the spasms started to return again after around six weeks. I let it go for a few months, as I thought they would eventually settle down and go away. I went back to the Professor in June 2018 to get another MRI and, lucky me, he found another compression. This one though was deeper in my Brain Stem, though, and in an awkward position. He informed me that it would be a much harder procedure. He agreed that he would give it a go, but that, if it looked like it was too dangerous once in, he would stop the operation, call it off and that would be it.

So, now I'm back on the Botox shots every three months, which I dread as I get around eight shots in and around my right eye as well as in my forehead, chin, and cheek. The shots into the corner of my eye are a terrible and painful feeling. The Neurologist that does them is specialized in doing these shots to Hemifacial Spasm sufferers and does a great job. He gets me great results every time.

These days I still continue to suffer with the "drums" beating in my head when I sleep. I roll around all night trying to lie in the correct position so I don't feel the spasms and drums.
I am not done with this journey. I will be going to see The Guru of MVD's, who is in another city, in Sydney, Australia. I just need to build up the courage once again to go through with it. Until then, I will keep living with these spasms and ruining every photo that I take with my beautiful family.

Denise Starkey

My name is Denise. I'm 57 years old, from the United Kingdom. This is my Hemifacial Spasm story.

I probably noticed the spasms around nine years ago. It initially began with just a flicker in my left eye. My GP said it was stress, as I was coping with several difficult things. I was told that I should "go somewhere remote and scream to let it all out!!"

The spasms gradually increased to the point that my cheek and mouth were both affected. I started receiving Botox injections every three months around the eye. I also chose to have an injection on my mouth once. The Botox froze my mouth so that I couldn't smile on that side. It looked like I had suffered a stroke. Then in 2012, I actually did have a stroke. It was a transient ischemic attack (TIA or mini stroke), but the doctors noticed my eye straight away. They asked questions about the spasms thinking that they were a symptom of the stroke. Over the next several years the spasms grew worse. I began looking on the internet and discovered the Hemifacial Spasm Facebook group. What a great bunch of people! The advice and compassion were second to none and everyone completely understood what I was going through. It was there that I discovered that MVD surgery was an option. My neurologist had not mentioned it to me before. He was supportive when I suggested the surgery to him and asked me to write about what impact the condition had on my life. I'm in the United Kingdom, so all of my health costs were covered under the National Health Service. This included everything from Botox to MRIs, surgery to aftercare.

I had my MVD surgery at a hospital in the Midlands, United Kingdom on May 22nd, 2018. I woke up spasm free, but then the spasms came back. My surgeon couldn't understand why the spasms returned, as the surgery had gone smoothly. Sometimes the nerve just needs time to heal, though. The spasms continued and became so bad that, in August of 2018, I had Botox again. It was right before the new school year, as I work as a school receptionist. I was very despondent, but everyone in the trusty Facebook group was there with their reassurances and rightly enough. I just celebrated the one-year anniversary of my surgery and I'm delighted to say that I am spasm free!

Looking back, I can especially realize how much affect this condition had on my life. I lost my self-confidence. I even grew out my fringe so that I could try to hide my eye. Sleeping was an issue as well. The spasms seemed to really come on strong when I would lie down. I also strongly disliked having photos taken, but I would force myself to do so anyway. I was not going to "not be there" when my grandchildren look back at their early years.

Now, though, it is wonderful to have what everyone else takes for granted; a smile and a calm face!

Darla OLeary

My name is Darla OLeary. I am 67-years-old and I live in New Jersey, USA. This is my Hemifacial Spasm story.

My Hemifacial Spasms began about seven years ago. It started with some twitches in my left eye, but I thought nothing of it at that time. I was under a lot of stress so I didn't know if that caused the twitches. Regardless, this continued for about 3 to 4 weeks. I still thought it was just stress so I started googling my symptoms. I was obsessed with trying to find out what this was.

I spent so many months trying to figure this out. In addition, my symptoms were getting worse. Finally, even though I'm not a doctor myself, I found my own diagnosis by using Google. It made sense to me! "Hemi", meaning half, and "facial", meaning face, and then the spasm. This is exactly what I had!! I finally got my answer. Google is an amazing tool!

I then called a neurologist in my area and he sent me for an MRI. At this time, I knew nothing about a FIESTA MRI or anything else regarding this condition. I didn't know about support groups either, like the ones on Facebook for Hemifacial Spasm sufferers. Well, of course, the MRI showed nothing. The neurologist was looking for tumors, I believe, and he seemed to know nothing about compressions, etc. So, I took his word to mean that I was fine.

I continued having these spasms just hoping they'd go away. I started getting acupuncture; however, I got nowhere with that. Finally, about two years later, I started Googling again. I swear I don't remember how I came upon the Hemifacial Spasm support group, but I found it!! I was so happy to see that other people have the same condition as me! I joined the group and, since being in this wonderful group, have gotten an abundant amount of information. I found out that there was a surgery for Hemifacial Spasms, which I didn't know about. I've made friends on this group, which I'm grateful for.

Last year, I made the decision to call a neurosurgeon in NJ who deals with Hemifacial Spasms. In fact, he's the only one in NJ that deals with this condition. Unfortunately, he's located pretty far from me, but I went with it. They told me, at his office, that I needed to get a FIESTA MRI first before the surgeon would see me. They sent me to a neurologist in the same building who suggested that I start with medication first. I didn't like the effects of the meds so I stopped taking them. He then referred me to get Botox, which I didn't want so I declined. Next, he referred me to the surgeon down the hall from his office.

I went for a consultation with the surgeon. He told me that I definitely have Hemifacial Spasms! He told me he would do the MVD surgery, if I wanted it. I was so happy to think I would be rid of this awful condition so I agreed to the surgery.

On 1/21/19, I had the MVD surgery. My surgery went smoothly without any headaches or neck problems. I did develop a clogged ear about a month after surgery. I went to see my ENT for this and he put me on steroids, which resolved the problem about a week later. My MVD surgeon claimed the surgery had nothing to do with my ear issue, but I beg to differ. Sadly, at the end of the day, my MVD surgery was not a success. The surgeon told me to wait three months and he would perform another MRI to see if, possibly, the pads had moved or he had missed something. The MRI showed nothing different. The pads were in place. He said that he could do another MVD surgery but I could lose my hearing if he had to go up past my ear. I didn't want that so he referred me back to a neurologist down the hall who specializes in Botox treatments for this condition. On July 3, 2019, I had my first Botox injections. As of now, the Botox seems to be helping me. If for some reason the Botox stops helping me, I have decided to seek a second opinion at the end of this year. I have a copy of my MRI disc and will forward it to another well-known surgeon in Pittsburgh for another opinion. I'm trying to avoid going to Pittsburgh, though, as it is too far for my husband to drive me and I'm certainly not going by myself. So that is my story as of today, as my journey continues.

Jenny Sander

My Name is Jenny Sander and I am 61-years-old. I live in Toowoomba, Queensland, Australia. This is my Hemifacial Spasm story.

I'm a teacher by profession, having taught early childhood classes - Preschool, Prep and Primary grades since 1978. I'm also single and an only child to Australian parents. I was born in London, England while my father was studying there in the late 1950s. My parents lived in England for six years before coming back to Australia with me when I was 2.5 years old.

My Hemifacial Spasm story began approximately 16 years ago when I was teaching a Preschool class in Brisbane, Queensland. From memory, I believe I noticed the first slight tremor and annoying but tiny pulsing twitch in my left upper eyelid, on and off from the beginning of 2003. It's been just over 16 years ago now. It stays in my mind because that year I had just returned to Preschool teaching after a period of leave. That little twitch was annoying, but I wasn't overly concerned and just told myself it was because I was tired, always busy at work, and dealing with some extra family issues at home. I watched and waited for my twitch to go away, but it did not. In fact, it never really stopped. Even as I was falling asleep and waking up in the morning it would continually be there, but only in my left eye. A bit weird I thought.

Taking leave from teaching two years earlier, I had tried my hand at a few other jobs, just for the challenge of doing something new. I worked in a very busy call centre dealing with insurance claims; I worked in a travel agency as I love travelling and had done a lot of overseas travel in previous years; I was a relief teacher travelling throughout the large Toowoomba school district and outlying Darling Downs country areas; and I even worked as a Bureau of Statistics Census collector which provided great exercise and a sore back in the days before online Census returns! I enjoyed meeting and talking with new people and, for a short time, relished the challenge of new and varied work experiences.

During this leave, I stayed with my parents at our Toowoomba family home, as my Dad had developed some health concerns after suffering a minor stroke several years earlier. Thankfully, he had made a full recovery. However, after retiring from his very busy profession as a General Surgeon and Specialist Urologist, he began to show signs of other health issues. He was diagnosed with Chronic Lymphatic Leukaemia and by 2006 he was found to have the early stages of Vascular Dementia. This came as a complete shock to me, as I was very close to my father and had always considered him to be invincible! As a compact family of three we set about coping with this news the best we could and took each day as it came. Roles were reversed fairly soon and I was beginning to feel that I was the parent figure in the relationship.

Life was pretty stressful as a result, with Dad needing more and more care and assistance. My eye twitch began to escalate in intensity and moved down to include the area underneath my left eye. I would twitch rapidly and have no control of the movement, which was very annoying and tiring. Sometimes it would pause for a brief minute and then start again for no apparent reason. Smiling, face to face conversations and nervous tension would set it off regularly and mostly it was constant.

Naturally, I thought this problem was due to the added stress of dealing with Dad's health decline. My Mum also had mobility issues and at the end of my leave she had undergone surgery to have a double hip replacement due to bad arthritis pain. I needed to be around for both my parents now, so I switched to part-time teaching to give me the chance to also help out at our family home in Toowoomba. Having no brothers or sisters, and all our close family members at opposite ends of Australia or overseas, I strongly felt I needed to be there.

Between 2003 and 2006, my life consisted of living half the week in Brisbane to continue teaching, and the other half week driving back to Toowoomba, a 1.5 hour drive each way, to stay at my parents' home and help with whatever was needed. This included housework, shopping, transportation, paying bills, gardening and coordinating doctor's visits and medications.

Around 2005 my blood pressure was tending to be high whenever tested, and I had been treated for some time for a hypothyroid (low thyroid) condition. As a result I had symptoms that meant I was constantly tired, experiencing hair loss, always feeling cold, and suffering with dry skin and hair most of the time. Typical symptoms of low thyroid function. My GP prescribed blood pressure medication and a beta blocker to regulate the heart fibrillation I was also getting more often. I was given thyroid hormone (Thyroxine) to take daily and now have to continue this for life.

After starting the blood pressure tablets, my more obvious eye twitches became less prominent for a few months, but as work at school picked up, they soon returned as badly as before. At school, I was becoming quite self-conscious when talking to colleagues, parents and of course the children. My pre-schoolers wouldn't hold back and were very quick to point out my "funny twitchy eye" on a regular basis. Thanks, kids!

Parent meetings, too were an ordeal. At interviews, or when I would have to speak to a group of parents at a meeting or give a presentation, I felt odd, looked odd and could never predict or control what my face would do at any given moment, particularly if I was feeling anxious. I felt that I looked unprofessional and nervous, and I worried that parents would be concerned that I was not up to the job. Of course the parents were lovely and supportive, but I was anxious and unhappy about my problem.

While in Toowoomba, I went to see an ophthalmologist to see if my twitches were an eye issue. I wanted to rule out any sinister causes such as a tumour or growth, but thankfully the main results were all clear. The only test out of the ordinary was a field vision test that I had to take twice. In both tests it showed that my left eye (my HFS side), was poor in seeing a flashing light to the sides of a fixed middle point. My right eye was perfectly normal. My ophthalmologist suggested it could be a neurological issue instead. I decided that, if things worsened, I would see a neurologist for further tests.

By 2006, I had had enough and finally asked my GP for a referral to see a Neurologist in Brisbane where I was teaching. I made an appointment with a senior Neurologist in Brisbane and took my Dad along for the ride, as despite being pretty frail now; he was concerned about my condition. He had started to show significant deterioration mentally and even though he was struggling to cope, mentally and physically, he still knew enough to be equally concerned for me.

The neurologist was lovely, well respected, similar in age to my Dad, and very experienced. He gave me a thorough neurological examination and ordered a MRI scan to rule out any serious concerns. I was relieved when he told me that the scan showed nothing really serious. There was no brain tumour or likelihood of any condition like MS (Multiple sclerosis), although I did have some small hyper intensive spots in the brain white matter that he called lesions. He said that nearly everyone has some of these, particularly as we age, and that they need to be watched if I had further issues with the twitches. He believed that he could just detect a slight compression (an artery touching my facial nerve), but suggested if I had future problems, that I should see a neurosurgeon for further advice. As an older Neurologist, he was about to retire, so he recommended that seeing a neurosurgeon would be the next step if I was troubled anymore. He also suggested watching that my diet was healthy, taking some folic acid supplements and that losing some excess weight would be ideal. A challenge that I'm always working on!

He did not believe medication would really help, and said that Botox may relieve the symptoms if I wanted to follow that path. I was reluctant, as I saw this as masking my twitches and spasms and that then I wouldn't know if they were progressing or remitting. He told me that as a last resort surgery was possible, but there were significant risks to hearing, balance and even vision, so it was not something he would recommend at this early stage. All I knew was that Hemifacial Spasm was starting to strongly affect my confidence socially and making my interactions with other people miserable.

I would avoid all photos whenever possible. As soon as I tried to smile it would set off a series of spasms, so school photos became very difficult and embarrassing. Once my teacher aide took an informal photo of me with a group of children. I thought I was smiling ok, but when I saw the photo, I was horrified to see that my mouth had drooped and I looked like I had had a stroke. That really hit home, and I visited another Neurologist to confirm I hadn't in fact had a stroke. All was okay thankfully, but I was still pretty miserable and becoming very depressed about the situation.

In 2007, I was asked to go back to a full-time teaching load as the new Prep Curriculum (1st formal year of school in Queensland) was being introduced into our State Schools, and Preschool was phased out. I became much busier at work and consequently so did my spasms. For that year, I spent each weekend travelling backwards and forwards to Toowoomba. At the same time, my father's health continued to deteriorate rapidly.

By 2008, Mum and I realized that we could no longer manage my father's care safely at home, and his GP advised us to place him in a local aged care secure Dementia ward. This was one of the hardest things we ever had to do, and we truly went through a period of mourning and misplaced feelings of guilt at not being able to continue caring for my Dad at home. For the next two years our lives were dominated by almost daily visits to the Dementia unit, and ensuring Dad's needs were being met. As time went on my spasms intensified, and Dad lost his speech, independent movement, his knowledge and memories.

While this was going on, I visited a Brisbane Neurosurgeon in 2010 to further discuss my spasms and possible treatment. I had another MRI and yet again he confirmed my condition was Hemifacial Spasm. He confirmed that he could see an area where he suspected a section of artery was pressing against my facial nerve. Again, he recommended Botox as the best treatment, and said he would not recommend surgery in my situation, as it was too risky. By now, I was certain there was no sensible alternative and nothing I could do other than ongoing Botox treatments. He stressed that if something went wrong during or after surgery I would find it difficult to care for my parent's needs. Reluctantly, I dismissed the idea of surgery as a possible solution.

Parents of young children often feel the same responsibility and dilemma, in choosing the surgical option. In any case, I put the idea to rest as it all seemed impossible and hopeless.

From 2010 – 2012, I took my long service leave and was allowed to access my remaining sick leave, which had accumulated over my 30 +years of teaching, as I was now caring for my Mum. I did some relief teaching but was mainly kept busy with carer duties and tending to our considerable size garden of two acres. I got to work weeding, pruning, removing and planting trees and shrubs and I found it to be therapeutic and a great stress relief.
Sometimes I overdid it and felt the consequences, particularly so when I had a nasty fall down a steep slope in our garden, and broke my right ankle. This was just after a major flooding episode in our town, when the ground had been saturated and was still muddy and slippery. So in 2011 I had my first major surgery to repair and pin my right ankle bones that had separated and fractured when I fell. Great! Something else to spur my facial spasms into overdrive. It seemed I just couldn't win.

Recovery took quite a few months, but Mum and I did a great job of managing and muddling along together until I was back on my feet again.

In May 2012, my dear Dad passed away, after a long battle with his Dementia and Leukaemia. At the end it was a relief he was no longer suffering the many indignities that Dementia brings. I managed to write and read the eulogy at his funeral, but was glad that the spasms were pretty low key that day and not too obvious to everyone. I think Dad may have had something to do with my unusually calm face on that day!

Life went on with just Mum and me, and finally I decided to take my Mum for a trip to Melbourne to see her sister for the first time in many, many years. Of course, there were the usual photos and I dreaded seeing my distorted face as I tried to control the rapid eye winking and spasming cheek that is often typical of Hemifacial Spasm. I felt self-conscious and could see others were puzzled by the change in my appearance as I tried to explain why I was constantly twitching and spasming. I was becoming truly fed up with doing nothing, so I resolved to reconsider and research having Botox Injections as soon as I could find an experienced doctor willing to treat me.

My salvation came in mid-2017 when I decided to join Facebook for the first time to keep in touch with our distant cousins and friends, and also to continue researching my Hemifacial Spasm condition. Being out of my normal work environment had isolated me socially and I wanted to reconnect with family and friends again.

One November night something prompted me to do an internet search on HFS information, and I stumbled across three Facebook support sites for people with Hemifacial Spasms. I signed up to be a member of each one and posted a question that ended up changing my life for the better.

My question was: "Can anyone recommend an experienced Neurosurgeon who regularly performs MVD (Microvascular Decompression) surgery for Hemifacial Spasms?"
Within hours, I had received several responses and most people highly recommended the Sydney surgeon that I chose for my surgery in May 2018.

I was so relieved I had found a supportive community of fellow Hemifacial Spasm sufferers, and reading about their experiences and feelings made everything less stressful. Here were people like me dealing with the same problem, a rare neurological condition. I began to think I may just have some hope of finding a permanent cure for my Hemifacial Spasm symptoms.

Being able to contact other group members who had already undergone MVD surgery and discuss their feelings, experiences and recovery was just what I needed. I began to get excited. I couldn't wait to make plans to travel to Sydney to see the surgeon I hoped would agree to operate. I asked my GP for a referral and took along my old MRI scans and reports for reference.

When I went for my first appointment with my surgeon, I was booked to first undergo a new MRI as my old scans were from 2006 and 2010. Following that, I met with my surgeon and nervously described my problem. I didn't need to really. My face was spasming away furiously and I was grateful it was putting on a show, as I wanted him to see the full condition I had been dealing with for the last 15 years. He immediately offered the comment; "Hemifacial Spasm?" and I nodded in reply. He listened intensely to my words and, for once, I really felt that this doctor understood my problem and concerns and may be able to help. He showed me on the MRI scan where I had a very obvious "U shaped" compression loop which was an artery pressing on my facial nerve. He described the surgical procedure simply and also inquired if I had ever tried Botox. I explained my thoughts on not wanting a temporary fix as I had turned 60 and was concerned about damage to my nerve if I postponed my surgery any longer. I also had age concerns for being a suitable candidate for surgery, but my surgeon reassured me that that was not a problem in my case.

He proceeded to explain that the MVD surgery involves undergoing a craniotomy whereby an incision would be made behind my left ear. A matchbox size opening would then be made through the skull to gain access to the offending artery/arteries that were making contact with the facial nerve. Once located, he would reposition the artery/arteries away from the facial nerve and cushion with a Teflon pad to prevent the nerve and artery from making contact.

Basically, the compression shown in the MRI scan was rubbing against my facial nerve causing it to be continually irritated, thus causing the twitches and spasms. As the myelin sheath coating of the nerve was deteriorating the nerve was becoming more and more irritated.

It all made sense to me from my previous research on this condition, and was what I suspected was the problem that I had developed. The cause is not really known, but it is likely I had been born with my artery/arteries positioned too close to the facial nerve. With age, the arteries had twisted and increased in size to where they had begun to pulsate and rub up against the facial nerve right near the brain stem. I told myself that I basically needed to fix a short circuit in my brain, and my neurosurgeon was the electrician!

I think the deciding factor came for me when I asked, "If I choose to live with my spasms and do nothing, will the spasms get even worse over time?" My surgeon nodded and confirmed what I probably already knew to be true. The spasms are usually progressive and would most likely become more intense. I was certain I could not endure them getting worse and possibly becoming tonus spasms that can distort your face for minutes at a time. No, I was certain that I wanted the surgery.

The surgeon said my compression looked fairly straightforward to fix, and then gave me the risk percentages for any problems such as hearing loss, stroke, vertigo, recurrence of spasms, etc. As head of the neurosurgery department, he was very experienced in MVD surgery and I felt 100% confident that he had the skills, knowledge and experience to fix my problem. His kind and gentle manner was reassuring and I was sure I wanted him to perform the surgery, as long as he thought he could fix my spasms for good. I was terrified he would have some reason to reject the idea of surgery, but when he agreed he could operate, I had never felt so relieved and happy. I was getting my life back at last!

Six weeks later I was flying down to Sydney solo for my MVD operation and I was full of optimism. Amazingly, I did not feel overly nervous. I was more excited as the time drew near and sure that I was doing the right thing. I was admitted to the hospital at 3:00 p.m. the day before for my final pre-op tests. This included Chest X-ray, ECG, and CT scan and prepared with stick on fiducial markers (circular white discs that look like lifesaver lollies) on my head and scalp. This was to help the surgeon digitally navigate my head once the operation was underway.

My surgeon visited me the night before to reassure me all would be well, and that my operation would be the first of the day at 7:00 a.m. He smiled at me and said he was going home to have a good night's sleep in preparation, but I knew I'd be pretty much wide awake most of the night! I think I may have had two hours of proper sleep before I was up at 5:00 a.m. to shower and put on my compression socks in readiness for the wardsman to wheel me down to theatre.

I was ready and waiting for the show to begin when the anaesthetist arrived at 6:00 a.m. to send me off to sleep before I was wheeled into the surgical theatre. I never did get to see inside those doors, which was a little disappointing, but probably very wise for my blood pressure I think!

The next thing I remember was waking up in the darkened room of ICU with nurses adjusting my IV Drip. I felt neither pain, nor headache and just laid there thinking "I wonder what time it is." Nurses came and went and asked me how I felt. How did I feel I thought? Wow, I felt great and, for a while, completely forgot about the spasms as I was taking in my surroundings. I could hear the moans and groans of other patients and muffled conversations, but I was too busy looking for a clock on the wall to see how long I had been in surgery. To my surprise it was only 11:00 a.m. I relaxed back into the bed thinking, "It's all over and I'm not twitching". I never expected it to be immediate relief, so I was feeling wonderful. Not long after, the surgeon and his registrar arrived to check on me. He pointed out the fact that I wasn't having spasms and questioned how my hearing was feeling. I had a slightly clogged ear sensation, but not bad at all and my hearing was perfect, just as normal. That was a great realization, as hearing loss was a real concern. My only problem was an extremely hoarse voice that took a while to resolve, but was back to normal eight weeks later.

I was very thirsty and asked if I could have a drink of water but was only allowed ice chips. I gently swallowed, as I had been warned that swallowing may be difficult after surgery. However, all was good and I suffered no pain, sore throat or swallowing problems.
The nurses tried giving me some pain relief despite the fact I did not seem to be in any serious pain as yet. I had just maybe a slight tension headache across my forehead occasionally. I was thrilled!

The elation ended for a bit when I was given some strong opioid drugs and promptly vomited them both up. Even Panadol was not my friend for a while and I spent two days not eating as a result. On the way back to the general ward I was taken for another CT scan and then I was wheeled back to my comfortable ward room to rest and recover.

After two days, when I was starting to eat again, I felt well enough to ask my surgeon about the details of my operation. He told me that everything had gone to plan, and that despite seeing one obvious compression on the MRI Scan, there were in fact two compressions discovered causing the problem. One smaller compression was hidden behind the more obvious loop compression noted on my MRI Scan. My surgeon was able to relocate both compressions away from the facial nerve (VII Cranial Nerve), and he inserted a Teflon pad to cushion the area between the artery/arteries and nerve. He also told me that my compressions were located low down and pressing on my brain stem.

He confirmed my suspicion that not all compressions are detectable on MRI scans and that sometimes they are only fully revealed during surgery. He assured me that I should have no further problems once the nerve was fully healed. To assist in nerve healing he recommended I take Vitamin B12 during my recovery.

I spent the next 10 days in the hospital resting so that I was in the best possible condition for returning home. I needed to be ready to resume my regular carer activities for my Mum, so I chose to stay a bit longer in hospital. Normally others would stay about 6-7 days.

The nurses, doctors and physios were great and very attentive. I couldn't have asked for better treatment or attention to my needs. My surgeon visited daily and answered any questions I had. I looked forward to these visits and the reassurance they gave me. I felt safe and lucky that I didn't have any real problems or issues other than my hoarse voice. My iPad came in very handy for messaging friends and family as phone conversations just weren't possible without my normal speaking voice.

On my 10th day, I was discharged after my stitches were removed by the nurses. I had previously undergone another CT scan and Doppler scans on my legs to check for any blood clot complications. All was good so I was able to pack up for home. A friend collected me from the hospital, as I had quite a bit of luggage (I always over pack). We stayed in a local motel for one further night to make sure I was okay and flew back to Queensland the next day. My friend had been keeping an eye on my Mum while I was away and was a wonderful support person, encouraging me all the way. In fact, his youngest son has the same Christian name as the Surname of my surgeon, so we figured that this was the best of omens for a positive result.

We were right, of course! My recovery at home was smooth. As the weeks progressed, I felt better and better. On Day four post-op, while I was still in hospital, my spasms disappeared completely. By Week two, I was pretty much back to normal activities around the house, but I did tire very easily. I rested when I needed, took things slowly, but was able to function really well. I made sure I was careful to avoid bending over and lifting heavy items for the first month or two. By Week three, I was driving again and travelling short distances to the chemist or local shops and I felt wonderful. I was keen to share my story and managed to bore a few people with the finer details. It was a great feeling to have a face to face conversation again, without needing to look away. I could look people in the eye again with no fear of my face misbehaving. It was liberating and so wonderful to be free of the previous anxiety I had endured for 15 years.

In many ways, I have been extremely lucky that my condition developed so slowly over the 15 years, giving me time to research my issues. In talking to others I realized that the progression can be much faster and more severe in a matter of weeks and months. I am so very grateful that I found the Hemifacial Spasm support groups online. It was they who helped me to decide on a surgical solution to my problem and recommended my very talented surgeon. I continue to say to myself and others this has been the best decision I ever made for myself.

I am now very happy that my life is back to normal and that I am still completely free of those horrible spasms, twitches and facial distortions that made my life so miserable. I'm delighted that I have just celebrated my 12 month anniversary of my surgery on the 16th of May, 2018. I feel very confident that the Hemi-facial Spasms will stay away in the future. However, should they return for any reason I know an excellent neurosurgeon who can help and guide me. For that, I will be forever grateful.

Jane Winlow

My name is Jane. I'm 36-years-old and I live in the United Kingdom. This is my Hemifacial Spasm story.

It all began in February 2016. I was renovating my home and one of the jobs was to knock up all of the tiles on the ground floor, using a pneumatic chisel. This took about a week and was long, hard work. During this week, my left eye began twitching. We all know the twitch. The one you get when you are tired or run down. Fast forward a couple of weeks and the renovation was going well and my DIY input had slowed down, but the eye twitch was still there and pretty constant all day long. It was irritating, but I just kept saying it would "go away" and being a tough geordie lass, who doesn't like bothering doctors, I just put up with it.

After three months the twitch was still there, every day, all day and my husband insisted I visit the GP. It was a locum doctor who suggested a number of possible causes; coffee intake, oily eyelids or tiredness. He suggested three weeks with no caffeine and a visit to an Optician. I followed his advice and cut out coffee. However, my eye was still twitching. The Optician was amazed when I went to see him. He had never seen anything like it and referred me to a Neurologist.

My first visit to the Neurologist was at the end of May 2016 and she could see the twitch and also pointed out other areas that were twitching like my eyebrow, my cheekbone and further down my cheek. She administered Botox to me and made an appointment to have a MRI to rule out possible tumors and Multiple sclerosis. During this appointment, she did not have any suggestions as to what it could be. Well, Botox helped a little. The twitching was less intense, but was never gone completely. The Botox also messed with my face. I was lopsided; my eye was constantly dry and couldn't close. Five months after my original twitch began, things took a twist. My right side began to twitch as well. It was constant, all day long unrelenting twitching and flickering. So now both sides of my face were doing it and I looked like I was having a fit. The results of my MRI came back and it was all clear so I made another appointment with the neurologist. During this appointment, she ruled out Hemifacial Spasm and stated "You can't get it on both sides. You're too young. It's impossible." So, she began googling. In the space of ten minutes of her googling, I was diagnosed with benign essential blepharospasm (BEB) (I pointed out that my spasms weren't in sync), Meige Disease (my mouth also must be involved and it wasn't), Blepharospasm and Oromandibular Dystonia combined; needless to say this didn't fill me with confidence. Again, I had Botox. This time I had it on both sides.

About four weeks after the Botox, I was eating when suddenly my mouth locked. It felt as though someone was winding it up from my temple bone and then my right eye slammed shut. This was my first tonus spasm. Not nice with a lump of soggy bread in my mouth. Bah! These spasms continued multiple times a day for longer and longer intervals. I felt like a freak and began avoiding social situations. During this time, I continued doing research on Hemifacial Spasms, which seemed to be the closest fit other than me having it on both sides. Another appointment with the Neurologist came and went. Again, more Botox, more googling, no diagnosis except to tell me again it couldn't be a Hemifacial Spasm. It was impossible to get it on both sides. I walked out of that with all faith in the doctors sapped, dreading having to live like this for the rest of my life. Still, in my gut I knew it was Hemifacial Spasms.

New symptoms began to arise. My eyes would spasm in time to music, like a human graphic equalizer. Certain songs and tones made them go crazy! My ear on the right side would click and I would get "seashell" noises. I couldn't go anywhere noisy; certain voices would make me spasm. I could no longer drive long distances or at night, my relationship was suffering, I couldn't concentrate with work and sleep was disturbed every night. It was wearing me down. I read about MVD surgery and found a Neuro Surgeon in Bristol who had great successes and experience. If anyone could either confirm or deny my Hemifacial Spasm self-diagnosis, it was him. I began collecting information on this particular surgeon, Hemifacial Spasms, MVD surgery and printed it all off. In December, I made an appointment with my GP and took him all of the information that I had gathered. I asked for a referral to see this particular Neuro-Surgeon. Two weeks later, I got confirmation that the Ccg had approved my funding to have an out of area referral.

In January 2017, I travelled from Northumberland down to Bristol to see the Neuro Surgeon and have a MRI. I was nervous. What if he said it wasn't a Hemifacial Spasm? What if it was something that there was no possible fix for? I can't even describe the relief I felt when he confirmed that he could see compressions of the facial nerve on both sides and that surgery was an option. I don't think anyone who hasn't experienced Hemifacial Spasm will ever understand why we are so happy to be told we are getting brain surgery! The Surgeon explained that Hemifacial Spasms can sometimes cause "Doppler Spasms" which affect opposite side, or the brain fluid can move around flowing better after MVD surgery. With that in mind, the Surgeon and I agreed that I would have the right side surgery first, even though that side started later. We decided this because the right side's progression was much, much quicker and tonus was very frequent.

I was on the MVD surgery waiting list between January and September. During that time, my original Neurologist wrote numerous letters to the MVD Neuro Surgeon disagreeing with him regarding his diagnosis. She also refused to do Botox on both sides of my face tell me "if you only need an operation on one side then you only need Botox on one side." I had my pre-op tests for my surgery and didn't get the expected results from the lateral spread. Panic set in! "That's it!" I thought, "The Neuro Surgeon is going to change his diagnosis." Instead, though, he consulted with another Hemifacial Spasm specialist in Asia who confirmed that the lateral spread response is only present in 80% of cases. "What do you want to do?" the Neuro Surgeon asked. The way I saw it was that I had nothing to lose. Worst case scenario would be that I still had spasms and a scar. I was going to be no worse off.

September came and I knew my date would be coming soon, but my beloved dad was terminally ill with cancer. My days were spent at his bedside and, one Friday afternoon, I got a phone call saying they wanted to do my operation on the following Monday. I had to refuse because I knew the end was close for my dad. I could never have left him and gone to Bristol. He died peacefully on Sunday afternoon. Somethings make everything else seem unimportant and being there for him was one of those things.

My operation was arranged for September 25th. I went down to Bristol with my husband who was suitably terrified whilst I only felt excitement; this could be it, the end of my bilateral Hemifacial Spasm journey. I had the easiest recovery possible. I had no pain, no nausea and awoke spasm free on both sides. This lasted for about four days, but I knew it was a good sign. I had two side effects from the surgery. The first was that cigarettes tasted vile, the second was so did anything sweet. This is gradually easing off now 2 years later. Speaking to my Surgeon afterwards, he confirmed everything was as he had expected and there were multiple compressions. However, the surgery had been complicated in regards to my hearing nerve. Per him, padding a compression like that would have made me deaf. This highlights the importance of hearing monitoring during the operation. He found a solution by moving my hearing nerve and gluing it out of the way. Also, because I didn't have a lateral spread response he had to use guess work to make sure the compression was padded enough to stop the spasms.

My at home recovery was uncomplicated and generally good. I tired easily and this lasted for months, but otherwise I have no complaints. My spasms on the right side were easing and, after four months, subsided pretty much entirely other than when I was ill or really run down. However, the same couldn't be said about my left side. It was getting gradually worse and the left side tonus spasms, which had started just before my MVD Surgery, were getting more and more frequent. I knew there was going to be more to my Hemifacial Spasm story.

About five months after my surgery, I had a telephone consultation with the Neuro Surgeon. He said that, because my left side hadn't resolved, he wanted to see me again. In July 2018, I went for a MRI down in Bristol again and was told the compression was still there and would need a left side MVD Surgery. Again, I was overjoyed! I knew how well my right side had worked. Less pre-op testing was needed this time, as we knew lateral spread test didn't work previously.

In January 2019 my date arrived. I had short notice, but was eager to have it done. I was booked for January 28th. We traveled down to Bristol by train and checked into the hotel on Sunday. I had the pleasure of meeting one of the other members of the Hemifacial Facebook group who would also be having surgery the next day. Meeting her was amazing! Finally, someone who knew what it was like and could genuinely empathize and understand what I was going through. Although our families understand and care, no-one knows how relentless it is and how much it impacts us until they've experienced that constant movement.

Later that day, back in the hotel, my husband's phone rang. It was the hospital calling to say that my surgery may be cancelled. An emergency had come in. I was devastated. You psyche yourself up for the surgery and the desire to be fixed is overwhelming. It sounds heartless to say, but at that moment I didn't care if someone was injured, I just wanted to be fixed. That selfishness subsided straight away and the logical me knew I had to listen to my own advice that I had dished out to many other members of our group time and time again. "When something happens it's because it's not the right time and everything happens for a reason." We agreed that I would still attend the hospital and be put on the reserve surgery list. As long as there were no more emergency cases, I should still be operated on. My Hemifacial buddy wasn't so lucky. On the bus on the way to the hospital she got the phone call to say her operation was cancelled. She did have successful surgery two weeks later and handled the delay brilliantly, using the same "everything happens for a reason" logic.

After the second surgery, I woke up in the recovery room and began twitching immediately. It was not the same and not as intense or continuous. I knew what to expect so it never phased me. Tea time came and they brought me some food, as I was up dressed and feeling fine. I went into the bathroom and suddenly my vision doubled and intense nausea swept over me and I began to vomit. I was given some anti-sickness medication and began to feel better. The next morning, the same thing happened again so more anti-sickness was administered. After that, the nausea subsided and I was eating and drinking okay. Again, my recovery was great and I was released from the hospital on Wednesday afternoon with orders to stay at the hotel for one night before travelling the seven and a half hour train journey home.

It's now four months post-op. My recovery has been great. This time around I had no exhaustion like the first time and seemed to have pulled myself around much quicker. I'm not spasm free yet, but there has been marked improvement and I know it's just a matter of time until I am. Speaking to the Neuro Surgeon after my operation, he explained that my left side was complicated because the artery dissected my facial and hearing nerve. Because of that, it couldn't be moved away and had to be padded as much as he could without my hearing being affected. He did say that if this didn't work then there would be very little more that could be done, but I know it will work!

For now, Hemifacial Spams is still with me. It's still controlling certain aspects of my life, but nowhere near what it was before the surgeries. I'm beginning to feel like me again. I will always consider myself as having Hemifacial Spasms. I'm one of a select few who are unlucky enough to suffer from a horrendously debilitating rare condition. However, lucky enough to have made fantastic friends and a support network that is not only supportive but knowledgeable, informed and who genuinely understand and care for one another.

Kim Puckett

My name is Kim Puckett. I'm 46-years-old and I live in Auckland, New Zealand. This is my Hemifacial Spasm story.

February 19, 2019:
You haunt me every second of the day like a practical joker, but you're never funny. You embarrass me, cause me discomfort and tiredness, distract me from thought and conversation, and disrupt my sleep, my relaxation and my quiet time. You are persistent and annoying. You cause frustration, sadness and despair. I try and quieten you with Botox, try and tell you to lay off and leave me alone, but you're still there, in the background haunting and teasing me. You're a bully, you never give up. I've been under the knife for four hours to try and rid you once and for all, but you only went away for six months; just long enough to give me hope. Like a cruel twist, like a knife in my back you returned. How could you? It's been eight years of my life chipping away at me, driving me crazy. I've tried my best and I've succeeded in living with you. You have become a part of my every waking moment. Your name is unfamiliar to most, no one talks about you, and no one can truly understand your horrendous nature unless they themselves are living with you. Your name is Hemifacial Spasm and on the 5th of March 2019 I am finally going into surgery a second time; hopefully for the last time and I'll be rid of you, for good. My original smile will come home to stay and not a distorted, twisted version. I will be able to look people in the eye again when I talk and I won't get the puzzled look back from people anymore thinking that something is not quite right with me. I will never have to mention your name again or hide away. This is my hope for all those suffering with this awful disorder. We have to be brave, strong, faithful and trusting to the surgeons who work their miracles. It seems it's the only way out for us.

This is my Hemifacial Spasm story.

I started getting Hemifacial Spasms when I was pregnant with my daughter who is now ten years old. It started off with fluttering eyelashes and twitching on my left eye. At that point, I saw a regular doctor then a Neurologist who immediately diagnosed me with Hemifacial Spasms. He sent me off for a CAT scan. The symptoms progressed over time to include spasms of my cheek and lifting of my lip. My eye would close completely or by half. This was 24/7 and totally random, but was also triggered by anything that increased my heart rate. I became increasingly aware of people noticing and staring and commenting. I became self-conscious, depressed and withdrawn. I avoided social situations and meeting new people. Things became very difficult. I went down the treatment path of Botox with mixed results. I then decided on MVD surgery after about four years of spams and after trying Botox for nine months.

The surgery went quite smoothly, but I had the initial headaches and the intense fatigue set in for weeks afterwards. My spasms slowly stopped completely but returned about seven months later. Not quite as bad, but different and more progressed. I had Botox injections until I felt that it wasn't really an option for me, as it just half masked the problem and didn't fix it. I feared that going for Botox every three months for the rest of my life, which made me look lopsided, would eventually weaken the muscles and make me look like I had a stroke. So, I decided enough was enough and booked in for surgery number two.

My second surgery was cancelled twice. This was an ordeal in itself. Every time a surgery was booked you were never sure if it was going to be cancelled at the last minute due to more urgent cases. This also occurred during a doctors' strike so I had to give up my business of house cleaning. I could no longer make commitments to my clients, as I never knew exactly when the operation would occur. In addition, I knew that I would not be able to drive for six weeks. This was a hugely stressful and anxious time in my life. This just added to the buildup of getting me emotionally ready for the operation each time. Plus, there were my children, who were very scared that I may die. It was awful.

On the second surgery, I had a less successful recovery. I woke up with complete hearing loss in my left ear, double vision, vertigo and then went on to have more complications.

I was sent home after about a week. Within days I noticed dampness at the bottom of the wound sight and went to A&E where it was discovered that I had a CSF leak. I was admitted back to the hospital where I stayed for another week. They re-stitched the bottom of the wound on two occasions. First, with local, but they didn't stitch deep enough. The second time I was advised that I needed at least two deeper stitches. Apparently, since I had a CSF leak local was too much of a risk to the brain so I was asked to do it without any pain relief, which I had to legally consent to. The pain was excruciating and traumatic to say the least, but it fixed the leak and I was sent home.

A few days later I noticed fluid coming out of my left nostril. This wasn't normal so I readmitted myself to the hospital to get checked out, as I suspected I could have yet another CSF leak. Samples given at the hospital never concluded anything and I developed flu type symptoms. After four days in the hospital with no answers, I signed myself out due to the frustration of it all. I just wanted to go home to get better.

I went home and, within 24 hours, my temperature steadily rose to 39 c. degrees accompanied by an extreme headache unlike any I had had since surgery. An ambulance was called, as it was the middle of the night and I have young children. So, off to hospital I went where I was found to have an infection somewhere in my body. They ruled out chest and bladder infections so I assumed it had something to do with the Hemifacial Spasm surgery. I was kept in the hospital for another week on antibiotics and then sent home. So, roughly, I was in and out of the hospital for a month.

Since the surgery, I have had balance issues, vertigo and, as I said, complete hearing loss in my left ear. I saw a hearing specialist who confirmed that it wasn't due to swelling or fluid. He suspects that the 8th cranial nerve was cut during surgery. I was told that the 8th cranial nerve deals with hearing, balance and sends the messages to the brain. So, to conclude, I am now permanently deaf in my left ear, I have ongoing balance issues and constant tinnitus in my left ear. My surgeon has advised that it may take up to a year for everything else to settle down.

When they went in for the first surgery, it was just my 7th cranial nerve that was compressed and they wrapped it. When they went in for the second surgery, he stated it was still in place and doing its job, but that I had a second compression involving both the 7th and 8th cranial nerves. This compression was very close to the base of the nerves where they both branch out. He could see that they were both already quite scarred and damaged by the compression. He suspected that my hearing was going to be compromised due to the state of things being so tangled up with the artery.

My spasms have more or less gone at this point. I still get the odd twinge and it is worse when I'm stressed, tired or anxious. I am personally weighing up whether the results were worth it, due to the hearing loss and tinnitus. I feel I have swapped one issue for another one. As my surgeon has explained, it's a "wait and see game" that I must play as nerves are tricky little beasts that take a long time to heal. A millimeter a week, I understand. So, I'm hopeful that I will get my balance back completely and loose the annoying constant ringing in my ear. It's just that my brain has to adjust to its new reality and its new senses. It just has to learn to make sense of it all.

To sum it all up this isn't a disorder that I would wish on anybody. It strips you of who you are, it takes away your peace of mind and your confidence. It's just a constant irritation and the only permanent way out is a risky operation. Like me, even that risky operation sometimes work or brings along another whole set of new problems. It's just a risk that you have to take to be willing to bring to end this horrible lifelong disorder. You just have to be brave.

Fabiola Teresa

All for You, Oh Most Sacred Heart of Jesus!

My name is Fabiola Teresa. I am 41 years old and live in Aguascalientes, Ags. Mexico. This is my Hemifacial Spasm story.

I am a consecrated woman; I think the term "nun" is best known to all. A nun's life takes place inside the convent between prayers, meditations, and community life. It would to here however be easy to live with Hemi-facial Spasms; the nuns of life are activated like me. We do not have a static life. We constantly have a change of work. This puts us out with different people, in different places and cultures. This was something that I enjoyed before my Hemifacial Spasms, but when my spasms became more noticeable, all I wanted to do was to hide so that no one could see me.

My condition began when I was 29 years old. I was the administrator of the school. I taught cate to young children. I was happy in my vocation, giving myself without reservation to the mission. I had confidence especially confidence in myself as a person. I could smile and talk with people until a strange and barely noticeable tick in my left eye appeared. My first thought was, "I'm too tired and stressed and it will pass." However, that did not happen. It appeared it was here to stay.

For five years, I searched for the name of my illness. I could find no doctors who knew of this condition. I tried homeopathy, acupuncture, naturopathic medicine, as well as medications for the nervous system. I underwent psychological treatment as well and nothing worked.

The Sisters of my Congregation attributed my symptoms to the fact that I could not control my stress. They thought that I had reached the limit of my nervousness and they wanted to help me by reducing my work and responsibilities. Not knowing the cause of what was happening to me, I started to believe that I really couldn't control my nervousness.

After five years of searching, a Neurologist told me that my condition was called Hemifacial Spasm, that it was idiopathic and that it was only controlled with Botox. Knowing the name of my condition gave me great joy. I was also glad to know that there was a physiological reason and that it was not my nerves. This led me to study my condition and I found that the most effective way to rid myself of spasms forever was to undergo MVD surgery. Before finally making that decision and reaching the operating room, 10 years of my life had passed.

The day of the surgery, May 11, 2017, I heard them call out to me "Wake up, Fabiola, wake up, we're done." They were the voices of the nurses who surrounded me on my stretcher calling out to me. I opened my eyes. The surgery that would return my smile was over. I was in a large recovery room, still connected to monitors. There was a large lamp that lessened the cold that I felt in my body as the effect of the anesthesia wore off. With a little effort, I managed to see the time on the wall clock. It was after two o'clock in the afternoon. I had been unconscious for more than 5 hours. The question echoed in my mind. "Did you find the compression? Am I finally cured?"

After a few minutes I felt the spasms returning. Even more so, the spasms had never really gone. In a matter of moments, all my hope fell apart. In my mind I decided what many people thought, that my condition was psychological. I gave in to the idea to those who said that I was too nervous, that I should control myself more and that I was not able to bear much pressure. I felt silly and a failure for undergoing a surgery that was not the solution. In that cold recovery room, I broke into tears. It was then, that in the middle of my tears and grief that I spoke with my God, to whom I had consecrated all my life. I told him that since with a disfigured face, I could not continue to serve him and asked him why he did not return me to my health?

Still sleepy from the anesthesia I felt that someone was next to me. It was Bety, my community sister. I stood dressed in a robe, cap and mask. She dried my tears and encouraged me by telling me that the surgeon had found the compression but that the spasms would take time as the nerve needed to heal. His words gave me some hope.

Two days after the surgery, a complication arose. A leak of cerebrospinal fluid kept me hospitalized a little longer. Long enough to know the world of pain caused by the disease, to know the laudable mission of doctors, of the nurses and also to make deep and solidarity friendships. Just as my spasms continued to accompany me, I experienced the presence of God who as a faithful sentry was with me in my prolonged vigils in that room. "It will ease." Those were the insistent words of the good doctor. Like me he also hoped that the spasms would disappear.

It was very difficult to return to my Congregation. Although all the sisters showed me understanding and support, I had a deep sense of failure within me. I was ashamed that my spasms continued to sabotage my encounters, my projects, and my ministry.

Having spasms for 10 years had already wreaked havoc in my life. It had affected my self-esteem, my confidence, personal security, my interpersonal relationships, my work and my mission. Those 10 years were a continuous struggle for me. The spasms wanted to rule my life and they were beginning to. However, that apparent surgical failure eventually made me stronger. I decided to overcome and continue fighting to recover not only the smile on my face but the government of my life and my dignity.

The hope of waking up without spasms was still alive in me. Seven months after the first surgery, on December 12, 2017, I had another intervention. Before leaving home to go to the hospital for my second MVD surgery, my community sisters prayed for me. They told me that they loved me very much with or without spasms and that they would be waiting for me.

With confidence in God and the doctor I went back into the operating room. At the conclusion, the doctor said that the surgery had been a bit more complicated since the dressing placed previously was very much attached. After this surgery, my stay in the recovery room was longer and the effects of the anesthesia were stronger. I felt very stunned, everything was spinning, and I was very nauseous. When I woke up I knew that the surgery was not magical. I knew that only time would tell if this surgery had been successful. This allowed me to keep calm, although the spasms continued to accompany me. The recovery at home was slower as well. It now took me more than a month to drive again. My steps were very slow and my ear was slow to return to normal. The spasms persisted.

Three months after the second surgery, my doctor told me that it was necessary to be operated on a third time. He said that he did not give up and that I had all the physical conditions to try a third surgery. Before deciding to go forward with the third surgery, I got a second opinion from another surgeon. This surgeon is recognized worldwide for his success in MVD surgery. He saw the compression in my resonance and said there is a 90 percent chance that could make me spasm free. At the time of this writing, I have not been able to have the third surgery.

After two surgeries I have achieved about a 30 percent improvement in my face. The feeling of failure continued to persist but this has made me a stronger woman, I decided to get up and not let the spasms rule my life. It is not very easy for me. Things are not easy such as: reading aloud or saying a few words in public, meeting new people, having a conversation, smiling in the street, giving a class, presenting myself to a group of children or teenagers or sometimes even crossing an avenue, for me is a challenge. Most of the battles I win and the others I still run away from.

There are many people who do not understand how this condition can be so important. Even though it does not directly endanger life, or cause physical pain for most. Sometimes I do not understand it myself. What most people don't understand is that this condition hurts you on the inside. It makes you withdrawn; it isolates you, and destroys your self-confidence and self-worth. However, worst of all is that most people live in solitude and in the silence.

In my heart is the desire to not have spasms. I want to be well physically. I do not want to hide my face. It is my desire to continue serving God in my vocation with greater freedom. I also thank God that the spasms have revealed to me the strong and tenacious woman that's within me. I am certain that he is doing great things, that I am in his hands and that the path will soon be clear.

Karrie Ward

My name is Karrie Ward Martinez. I'm 60-years-old from Sand Springs, Oklahoma, USA and this is my Hemifacial Spasm story.

The spasms started about 2008. They were gradual at the beginning, starting around the eyes, but got worse as time went on. I was under a lot of stress and contributed my spasms to that. I finally asked a nurse friend of mine who she recommended I speak to about the spasms and she gave me the name of a Neurologist. He was an older man, but I trusted my friend's judgement. The first time I saw him, he sent me for an MRI of my head, looking for possible tumors. He said it came back normal and then sent me to an ENT. He reviewed my MRI and said I had a bad infection in my sinus cavity. YAH….I had found the culprit! However, after weeks of antibiotics, the spasms continued. The Neurologist started me on some "crazy" pills, due to my stress level. I took several different kinds with no relief. One day I called to make an appointment with him and his receptionist told me he no longer saw established patients, only new ones. WHAT??? That made no sense. She said "that's what I thought also, but hey, I'm just paid to answer phone, not question him."

I was then referred to another Neurologist by my friend. I asked him to not give up on me, that there was something wrong and we needed to figure it out. He assured me that he would not quit on me and that he would find the answer. By this time, my marriage had ended and I was hoping that, without the stress, things would get better. Unfortunately, this didn't happen. The Neurologist's diagnosis was that my nerve had caught a virus, which would take about five years to heal. In the meantime, he prescribed me medicine after medicine to give me relief. I even tried Botox, but that made my face worse than the spasms. I felt like my face was glued in place and couldn't move. I was not willing to try Botox again to see if the doctor could get it right. By the way, I went to a plastic surgeon for the injection of the Botox and not my Neurologist. No relief came and, after about four years, I quit taking all medications and stopped seeing the doctor. I had decided this was my fate, and nothing was going to cure me.

In 2014, I met and married a man, Jim, who happened to be a certified athletic trainer. He would lie in bed and rub my face trying to get the spasms to stop in hopes that I would get relief and sleep during the night. Nothing helped.

In early 2016, Jim came to me and said he found the problem on the internet. He told me it was Hemifacial Spasms and there was a surgery that could cure me. I was like "are you kidding me? Not one doctor could diagnose me and you found it on the internet!" We researched until we found a surgeon in Tulsa, OK that had experience with Hemifacial Spasms. I called and scheduled an appointment with him. I was thinking it would take weeks, if not months, to finally have the "official" diagnosis and then the surgery. Luckily, I got in relatively quick to see him. I assumed he would want me to have another MRI, but the minute he saw me, he diagnosed me as having HFS on the seventh cranial nerve. I asked him how he knew it was the seventh and he said that, with the fifth cranial nerve, I would have pain. Fortunately, I never experienced pain with my spasms.

We set up a surgery date for November 30, 2016. I couldn't wait. There was no hesitation or second thoughts for me. I was ready to get it over with. The surgery went well. I was so sick from nausea the first 24 hours but I was spasm free! I stayed in the hospital 3 nights and went home feeling pretty good. I took off work for three weeks. I have an office job, so it was easy to go back. I did work from home during those three weeks; probably more than I should have, but I would only work until I was tired, then I would stop.

I stayed spasm free for 18 months. In January 2018, I started having fluttering around my left eye again. The same way it started back in 2008. I didn't say anything to anyone as I was hoping it was just a temporary thing and would go away. It got worse over the weeks and drifted down my face. The first of May, I decided to go back and see the surgeon. Without performing a MRI, he agreed it had returned and surgery was needed. We scheduled May 14, 2018 for my second MVD surgery. This one was almost identical to the first one. My nausea was worse, which I didn't think it could be. Every time I was given medicine, either by mouth or by IV, I threw up. I have no idea what triggered it. I had to stay in the ICU for two nights this time due to the nausea and not being able to keep anything down.

I'm happy to say I am spasm free today. I did, however, lose my hearing in my left ear after the second MVD surgery. Would I do it again knowing that I would lose my hearing? Yes, it's definitely better than the spasms. My prayer is that I never have Hemifacial Spasm on the right side of my face. I'm not sure I could/would chance losing my hearing in right ear and be completely deaf. I would just have to deal with the spasms.

My story has a happy ending. I feel sorry for those who I read about who say surgery didn't help or who were told surgery was not an option for them. My best advice would be to find a Neurosurgeon who specializes in Hemifacial Spasms. From my experience and what I read from others, it seems Neurologists are not trained a lot in this area and it surprises me. Since being in a support group on Facebook, Hemifacial Spasms appear to be common around the world.

Brenda Kyne

My name is Brenda K. I'm a 58-year-old single mom from Northern California. This is my Hemifacial Spasm story.

It started with a tiny, barely noticeable pulsing under my left eye that never stopped. It only progressed. I was under enormous stress at the time having to place my blind mother with dementia into a nursing home. Additionally, I was purging and semi remodeling her home to rent out. I attributed the spasms to the stress at first. Also, ironically, my career is in medical billing, although not in a hospital. Sitting in front of two computer monitors eight hours a day became extremely difficult with my eye closing and "bouncing".

Lucky for me, my doctor diagnosed Hemifacial Spasm immediately but basically said, "You don't want brain surgery". So, the only other option was Botox. The very unsympathetic male Ophthalmologist, who gave me my first series of injections, basically told me that I would have to "just learn to live with it" since it would not go away on its own. He said "You don't want brain surgery". I burst into tears immediately. I endured four series of Botox injections over the next 18 months, which just left me feeling like a stroke victim.

At this point, I begin to google "Hemifacial Spasms" and stumbled across the mention of this Facebook group for the condition. It saved my life!! I then started to learn about the journey of people with Hemifacial Spasm. I read so much that I decided, hell yes I DO want brain surgery!! I had to go through the insurance hoops of my HMO plan in Northern California. My next step was a Neurologist consultation. Another win! He was supportive and knowledgeable. He referred me to Dr. C, a top Neurosurgeon at a major University teaching hospital, about an hour away. Unfortunately my insurance denied the request saying that "Hemifacial Spasm is not painful or life threatening" and stating that I must see one of two Neurosurgeons that were also an hour away. It turned out that only one of them even performs the MVD surgery that I needed.

My consultation with this young, attractive surgeon went well and he ordered my MRI. He later called saying that he could see the compression and was willing to do the MVD surgery. Although he seemed confident, it turned out, that he had only done 11 of these MVD surgeries. After agonizing and consulting with this Hemifacial Spasm Facebook group, I wasn't confident with his lack of experience. Therefore, I declined surgery with him.

I then went back and searched the surgeon list in the files section on the Hemifacial Spasms Facebook group and found and selected Dr. B.A. Again, he was in a big city an hour away. He had also done many successful MVD surgeries. Although he was later in his career, he was wonderful, skilled and compassionate. I felt enormous confidence in him.

I had my first MVD surgery on August, 8, 2018. The surgery went well. After a three hour surgery, I awoke with a screaming headache, but was spasm free. I went home on day four with pain medication and a steroid pack. My only recovery complication was a mild case of Aseptic Meningitis which was cleared up with a second steroid pack. I was back to work full time after six weeks.

All was well and I felt great until I came down with a head cold a month later. The spasms returned back with a vengeance. The nonstop thumping had returned in my ear, no sleep, non-stop major spasms and increased tonus. As a single woman, I found myself being reclusive and extremely depressed. I contacted Dr. B.A, who immediately ordered another MRI. I returned for a visit and we looked over the MRI scan. He turned to me and said "I'm sorry, but there must be another compression that I couldn't reach. You will need to redo the surgery." However, he informed me that he did not do revisions since they were much more difficult. He referred me to Dr. C who was my first choice that my insurance originally denied!

I impatiently waited to see Dr. C, who looked over the MRI. He suggested repeatedly that I take time to carefully consider what he thought would be a very difficult surgery. He cautioned that a revision only had a 65% success rate and he asked me what it would mean to my life to have this MVD surgery. I told him that it meant everything to me and that I did not need time to consider. I was absolutely ready to get started. Dr. C said that he would have the Chief Vascular Surgeon, Dr. A.A, do the surgery with him.

Surgery number two was on March, 25, 2019. After the surgery, which took seven and a half hours, Dr. C came in to let me know that it was a very hard and complicated surgery. They ended up doing what is called a "sling procedure" on one artery, but then the monitor picked up another compression somewhere else. They had to locate that compression and place his preferred fluffier Teflon padding. The surgeon was also unable to locate any Teflon padding from the previous surgery. I only had a few small spasms for the first day which lessened to zero by day four when I left the hospital. My energy and sense of well-being returned more quickly this time despite the longer and more difficult surgery. My one unforeseen complication has been spinal stenosis and a nonstop burning pins and needles feeling in my lower leg and foot. This is related to two previously undiagnosed bulging discs in my lower back which were exacerbated by the extended period of surgery in the Mayfield clamps. At the time of this writing, I will be having my 2nd Epidural injection for that this week.

I hugged Dr. C at my post-op visit. I told him that he was my hero and that his team had given me my life back. It was so very touching to see how my happiness seemed to greatly affect him. When I asked if there were any activities to avoid in the future, his response was to go live my life to the fullest and not think about Hemifacial Spasm again. He is a truly a great man and it's been an amazing journey that I could not have done without the support of the wonderfully supportive fellow Hemifacial Spasm family.

Louise Walker

My name is Louise Walker. I am 40 years old and live in England. This is my Hemifacial Spasm story.

Where do I even start in writing about my Hemifacial Spasms? It's impacted each and every part of my life, from home and relationships, work, emotional, social and everywhere in between. I've cried many, many tears but have also faced many fears and grown in strength as a person. It's been a very bumpy ride! I'll try and go back to the beginning.

Ten years ago I received the diagnosis of Hemifacial Spasms, but it had actually begun 2 years prior to that. My diagnosis is now bilateral HFS. In April of 2018, the left side of my face joined the party, but it was all those years ago that my journey started.

From what I can remember, I'd been having twitches for quite some time before I really paid much attention to them. I recall mentioning to people that my eye was bothering me, but I'd certainly never heard of Hemifacial Spasms. Like I did with most other stuff in my life, I found ways of brushing it off. Because everyone gets twitches, right? About a year after it started, my husband suggested that maybe I consider getting it looked at. It was beginning to annoy me and, when my hay fever flared, it was worse. My eye constantly felt gritty and dry. It was like having an irritating itch that you can't quite put your finger on to scratch it. I felt a bit stupid making an appointment for something seemingly so insignificant, but I needed to try and stop it. Plus, people were beginning to make pirate jokes and ask me why I was winking at them!

I booked my appointment and it's safe to say that it was a completely unremarkable. As soon as I began to talk, literally before I could even finish, the doctor told me it was stress and fatigue. I tried to explain that, whilst I am often stressed and fatigued trying to juggle a demanding and difficult job, three children and a life that's quite challenging, I certainly hadn't had twitches my whole adult life and stress wasn't a new thing to me. Plus, this had been going on for quite some time. The doctor reluctantly looked behind my eyes when I pushed a bit further and declared that he saw 'nothing sinister'. He concluded that I needed an eye test and to relax. As I've been wearing glasses since I was about 6 years old and had always had regular eye checks, I was pretty certain it wasn't that. However, I hadn't specifically asked my optician about the twitch, so I agreed that it seemed a sensible way to move forward.

Some months later, I made the appointment with my optician, only to be met with a similar, 'nothing sinister' diagnosis. She also concluded that I must be stressed and fatigued. I think I just gave up at that point. I didn't have the time or energy to deal with it. I was relieved that my eyes were healthy, but resigned to the fact that my face was rubbish. I felt pretty crushed and frustrated but, at that point, I think I still assumed it would probably go away. I mean, who has an eye twitch forever?! No one mentioned Hemi-facial Spasms. I'd never heard of it. I didn't think to Google it because why should I when medical professionals know best, right?

About 2 years later, (yes, I really waited that long and still didn't do anything!) the twitching became the more extreme spasm that I later became more familiar with. It couldn't be described as a twitch anymore. At this point, my confidence had taken a huge hit from the facial spasms and I was pretty low. Bit by bit, HFS had chipped little bits away from me as the months went by. But still I couldn't quite bring myself to fight another doctor to ask for some answers. I think it's quite a British thing to not want to make a big deal about something! I'd seen the doctor; she'd as good as sent me away. The optician had done the same so what did I know? I had no right to challenge that did I?! It's actually only recently, that I've changed that attitude and had the confidence to disagree and be assertive over my health care. The twitching was still localized to my eye, but it was definitely worse. I never told anyone how low it made me feel. It was only when I asked for the referral for surgery years and years later that I broke down and told people how it made me feel. Which, looking back now, makes me so sad.

Around that time, I fell and hurt my knee. I'd left it until it was really bad, as I generally do. I reluctantly made an appointment to see my doctor. At the end of the appointment, she stopped me and said 'Before you go, I see you have quite a significant eye twitch'. I remember that I kind of nonchalantly laughed it off. "Yes, I know, and I know what you're going to say; everyone gets them. Have I checked my eyesight? Am I stressed or tired?". "No", she said. "That's not what I was going to say". I sat back down with a great big sigh and she asked me to tell her about it. I talked and it was like a lid had opened and all these words were spilling out. How I felt, what I'd been going through, what I'd been storing up. That's the first time I heard the words, 'Hemifacial Spasm'. Her words were, "I think you may have Hemifacial Spasms and you need a MRI." I had a name and, for the first time in a long time, hope that I might find out what was happening with my face.

For two years after that, I managed well with Botox. My MRI had come back 'normal' and, so as Botox was the 'go to' thing in managing HFS, this was the option that was presented to me. For those two years, life really did go back to normal and I remember saying to my husband, "if it works like this forever, then I'm happy". However, at the end of 2015, it became apparent that the high dose of Botox that was then needed to manage the ever spreading and increasing spasms also left me with a very asymmetric face. I hated the monster in the mirror who stared back at me with a frozen Botox face, as much as I hated the monster who stared back at me when my spasms were in full swing. So with Botox no longer working and my face affected from eye, nose, cheek, lip, chin and neck, I honestly felt broken. More so than I ever had and I couldn't go on the way things were.

I had joined a support group online a couple of years before then and had seen this elusive brain surgery mentioned. Maybe I could have that too? So, after taking deep breaths, I asked my Neurologist about the surgery and was shot down with a big, fat, "no". He said "We just don't do that surgery in the UK and it's very dangerous". He then proceeded to prepare the Botox vial and I stood up and walked out of his office and never returned. I remember walking home from that appointment in the rain with tears rolling down my face. As much as I hated having to go back to my doctor, I felt I had no option but to book an appointment to ask about a referral for surgery. I honestly had no one left to ask and nothing left to lose. I didn't want a referral to a Botox clinic elsewhere and I didn't want to be brushed aside anymore. I didn't want to see another Neurologist. I wanted to see a Neurosurgeon who was a specialist in HFS. I wanted to talk about surgery.

I'm not an overly confident person at the best of times and the thought of having to ask an actual doctor for something is a pretty big deal for me. With this in mind and my anxiety high, I decided I needed to do some planning before I went in. I needed information. I needed to be able to explain who I wanted to see and why it needed to be them. I printed out the section from my surgeon's website on, 'how to refer'; in case my GP needed a little bit of a push, too. I wanted to know about my rights for referral and found an NHS document to back me up. I thought of all of the questions the GP might ask and how I would answer them. Then I decided I would just burst into the appointment and start straight away with, "Please can I have a referral. Thank you very much". I also decided to arm myself with a video. On the whole, my face was always badly behaved, but it could be variable as to which parts would spasm and how severely. So, I had spent a few weeks filming it at its worst.

I want to say that I very calmly presented my case to my GP, who reviewed all of my information before we then had a very mature discussion that led to her agreeing to a referral. However, what actually happened was I burst into tears, did big ugly crying, and amazingly had some kind of conversation where she agreed that it was appropriate for me to at least have a chance to speak to an expert. Being the incredible GP that she is, she told me that she would go home and draft a referral letter over the weekend. She explained that she would do everything she could to get me to the surgeon I had requested and that no news was good news. Walking home in the rain and the dark, all I could do was smile. I wanted to stop everyone I passed and tell them my news!

A week before Christmas, I got the best present ever. I got my appointment for 18.01.17. An MRI at 9am and a consultation at 10am was the very best start to the brand new year. That appointment was life changing. On that day I met the kindest, most empathetic and understanding Neurosurgeon. He assured me that he would sort me out and has supported me ever since. To cut a long story short, since then, I've had two MVD surgeries, a couple of other surgeries and a range of complications. I now have a left side where some days I have no spasms and when I do have them, they're so insignificant they don't even bother me. Surgery has been life changing and I'm forever grateful to the incredible skill of my Neurosurgeon. Whilst I have a bilateral diagnosis, surgery has put me in a place where I can manage.

What I haven't touched upon so far, is quite how significantly affected I've been emotionally by HFS. As a patient, if I could only speak about one thing to a medical professional about my HFS, I would want them to know how hard it is to live with. To not underestimate the impact it has on an individual. There is more than one way to feel pain and, just because it's not always physical, doesn't mean it can't still cut deep emotionally. HFS is socially isolating, debilitating, lonely and devastating. Make no mistake of that. Life, over the years, has been so full of difficulties in living with HFS. I have struggled and faced feelings, thoughts and situations that have been incredibly hard to deal with. Physically, it's been tough. My vision has been affected by the spasms, the aches and significant pain caused by my face just having enough. But emotionally, it's been unbearable. I've hidden in toilets and cried. I've had people asking me in front of my friends and family, what was "wrong with my face". I've had medical professionals dismiss Hemifacial Spasms as a 'minor inconvenience'. I've had one health professional declaring I had Tourette's. Trust me, I have hurt and I have cried.

However, I promise you, as tough as it's been; HFS in some ways has helped me grow as a person. I have learnt the most valuable lessons in empathy and understanding. If someone is 'different' it isn't for me to judge or question but to support and accept. I find myself drawn to people who face similar challenges to me; even if on the surface they appear very different. I have learnt just how much my friends can support me now that I have shown how HFS makes me feel instead of always brushing it off. Knowing that I don't have to laugh it off and pretend I don't care. I'm much more open than I was about how it makes me feel. I know that my family loves me, face and all, and that often they face the same fears as me as they also learn to deal with my feelings and struggles. I know now that I CAN face things and hold my head high. Do I often hide behind my hair and wish the ground would swallow me? Sure, and when the spasms were at their worst that was me most days. There are times where I sit quietly in meetings, in conversations, even when I desperately want to contribute and I still can't look people in the eye. I still look at the floor when I respond to someone's greeting on a bad day. But I can stand tall if I need to.

I guess to finish this (although I could go on forever) is the way that HFS has touched me the most. It's touched me in a way in which I never expected. I have met strangers who have changed my life in the most incredible way and been a part of me growing as a person. The one thing I have always known is how blessed I am, not in a religious way, I don't follow a faith, but in a 'the world is a wonderful place' way. The world is full of beautiful people and experiences everywhere you look. My life is by no means perfect. Aside from HFS, I've had trauma and I've had hurt, the same as everyone, but I count myself as one of the luckiest people alive. Importantly, I've also learnt that sharing my experience can sometimes help someone else come to terms with theirs. I really hope that someone, somewhere reading this might have a glimmer of hope that all will be ok, and that they aren't alone.

Finally, to those who don't have Hemifacial Spasms? I ask you, please be kind, be sensitive, be nice and above all, be accepting. Because we see you stare and we hear you whisper.

Samudyatha Bhat

My name is Samudyatha Bhat and I am 33 years old from Bangalore, India and this is my Hemifacial Spasm story.

First of all, I am a classical dancer in India so my face plays a big part in my career. My journey with Hemifacial Spasms started around 3 and a half years ago. My right lower eyelid started fluttering first. It would continue throughout the day. Worried, I went through the internet googling my symptoms. I then booked an appointment with a Neurosurgeon. The surgeon wanted to rule out the possibility of a vitamin B12 deficiency and asked me to take a blood test. The blood test report showed that my B12 counts were low. I was prescribed a vitamin B12 supplement for a month and that was of no use. Though my B12 count did increase, my right lower eyelid twitching had not stopped. It was then that my doctor said that it may be a Hemifacial Spasm (HFS).

Since the twitch was very mild, I neglected it. Then after a few months, the upper right eyelid also started twitching. I then met with a couple of other neurologists who suggested that I take Tegretol tablets to see if they would help. However, consuming Tegretol made me sleepy all the time and I begin to find it difficult to balance myself. So I had to stop taking the drugs. One of my friends, who had suffered from Bell's palsy, suggested to me that Ayurvedic medicines may help. So, I also tried Ayurvedic medicines next. Those medications would help me in reducing the twitching. However, the twitching returned once I finished my course of medication. By this time, my spasms had increased and had spread to my cheek, lips and neck as well. Both doctors had suggested that I try Botox instead of surgery which I declined.

I found myself in need of a good Neurosurgeon. After researching the doctors on my own, I found a Neurosurgeon from Pune who was an expert in MVD surgery. I made up my mind to undergo the MVD surgery. To get to the Neurosurgeon, I had to travel from Bangalore to Pune which was a 2.5 hour flight. My first visit with him he performed a MRI where he located the compression loop and told me that I was a candidate for the MVD surgery. Together, we set a date for the surgery.

The surgery was set for April 9, 2019. I arrived once again in Pune a day before my MVD surgery. My pre-op bloodwork was done, along with urine tests, x-rays and general fitness tests. My head was also partially shaved to prepare for the surgery.

On April 9th, 2019 I had my MVD surgery and woke up spasm free. However, on the 9th day post-surgery I developed facial weakness and was unable to move my face on the side on which the surgery was performed. The Surgeon assured me that I would recover. Luckily, after 6 weeks post-surgery I regained most of the facial movements and continue getting better every day.

Being an Indian classical dancer my facial expression matter the most. Due to the HFS, I had lost my confidence to perform on stage, which affected my life. I am happy to say that I'm still recovering now and will be able to continue to perform soon.

Angela Bond

My name is Angela Bond and I'm 69 years old and live in the UK. This is my Hemifacial Spasm story.

It started with a twitch…….

It started with a twitch back in 2004 when I was 54 years old. What did it do to me? Well, it didn't kill me but little by little it began to destroy my sense of self, my personality and some of my relationships. Others really didn't 'get it' and would tell me that it was nothing; this made me feel as if I might be going mad because it certainly felt like something to me. As time went on I began to feel a lesser person than others and would hide away from the world and withdraw socially. I gave up the job I loved and, with a degree of acceptance, I saw HFS as a punishment that I deserved.

I live near to Winchester in the UK and first developed an annoying little twitch in my right eye shortly after I met Gog (short for 'good old Graham'). For better or for worse, for him, he would later become my second husband. The obvious conclusion is that Gog caused it, but I don't think so. I'd had a turbulent few years and just when I was getting my life back on track, along came HFS. But enough about HFS, let me tell you about me………

I've always been a worrier and a stressy person. I can worry for England, Scotland and Wales. If I see an ambulance, I am convinced one of my children is inside. If I get a spot, it has to be skin cancer. When working as a social worker I could never leave even one piece of work until the next day or I would worry about it all night long. Get the drift? Yes, totally neurotic. My other failing is that I care too much; I feel everyone's pain as if it's my own, and that can be testing for me and others. I worry about people but thankfully I don't worry about housework, money or material possessions. I love gambling on the horses and I'm a prolific loser, but not in debt.

Anyway, the menopause wasn't a great time for me because, as well as having nasty migraines and joint pain, I went off my trolley. There I was with a good husband and three super grown up children, and I decided to blow it all. I blame it on the hormone replacement therapy they gave to me; nothing to do with me officer. But I've always believed that HFS was my punishment for messing up my family. I accepted the punishment without question and this perhaps helped me to cope with HFS and to never say 'Why me?'

I was luckier than some, because when I went to see my family doctor, she took one look at me and said 'You've got something called Hemifacial Spasm' (HFS). She referred me to an ophthalmologist at the local eye clinic and from there I was sent straight for Botox treatment. There was never any suggestion that I needed an MRI scan to rule out other possible causes. I started receiving Botox within a few months of first diagnosis. For those readers who do not live in the UK, I should point out that health services are free to all in the UK and we don't have to worry about insurance or anything like that. It's called the National Health Service (NHS) and was introduced in 1948. I've made good use of it and thank God that we in the UK are lucky enough to have it.

I remember asking the Botox nurse if she saw much HFS and she told me that it was relatively rare. She went on to say 'some people end up needing brain surgery'. What? Had I heard that correctly? I laughed this off as something that happened to others but certainly wouldn't happen to me. At this stage I didn't feel overly worried about my twitching and was optimistic that Botox would be the answer. Luckily I didn't have any clue that HFS was a progressive condition. I had no other points of reference at this time and didn't obsess about it; it really wasn't that bad, just an annoying intermittent twitch.

My first lot of Botox did limit the twitching but made one eye look bigger than the other. I asked if I could have a balance shot in the other eye but was told that the NHS couldn't run to this as it would be viewed as cosmetic. I quite liked the 'ironed look' of my right eye, but it was rather weird to look young on the right and old on the left. I felt a bit like Julio Iglesias, a singer who would only ever show the more handsome side of his face to the cameras.

It was around a year into my HFS journey that I got a new job as a hospital social work manager in the same Salisbury hospital where I had my Botox. I'd never wanted to be a manager, but I was flattered into doing it; big mistake. Up went my blood pressure, up went my stress levels and crazy went my spasms again. The mouth started to join in with the eyes and I was very self-conscious. I used to dread going to work and facing strangers and clinicians who I felt were judging me on my weird appearance. I felt more like the service user than the social worker and was sure that others saw me as mentally deficient. I would make a bit of a joke of it and explain that I wasn't winking at anyone, but I often felt the embarrassment of others when they averted their eyes or even started doing a sympathy grimace. After about 9 months I decided that I just couldn't do the job any more. I gave in my notice and returned to a less full-on role with a local carers' charity. There I met the dreadful Charlie who was enough to make anyone twitch! She was the boss's 19 year old daughter and was of the mistaken belief that I was for bossing. In your dreams Charlie, HFS or no HFS.

Quite unexpectedly, after changing my job, I went into full remission for a few months. I foolishly thought this was the end of HFS for me, but not so. We moved house and this brought the spasms back into full swing, with the mouth pulling badly up towards my eye at fairly regular intervals. My triggers would be tiredness, cold, toothpaste, eating, drinking, sunlight and any animated conversation or laughter. It was at about this time that I felt my personality ebbing away. I had to run a training course for new volunteer advocates and found myself apologising repeatedly for how I appeared. The standard response from others was always 'we can't even notice it' and for some reason this made me want to punch them. I was getting phenomenally tired with the strain of trying to fight my face at the same time as delivering a lively and interesting course. I used to be totally done in when I got home from work and when Gog spoke to me my heart would sink because all I wanted was quiet. I'd always been a noisy and talkative person but not so any more. Darkness and quiet were my comfort zones.

I started to research HFS on the internet and found out that, besides the usual cause of a compressed facial nerve, there could quite rarely be other more sinister causes. I was now in full blown neurosis and started sending away for every research paper ever written about HFS. Panic stations……. I went to a new GP and asked if I could see a neurologist. The doctor, who was about 12.5 years old and fairly fresh out of college, hadn't heard of HFS before and decided that I didn't need a neurologist. He prescribed Carbamazepine, an anti-seizure drug.

The Carbamazepine had the effect of making me feel hideously depressed and my blood pressure went through the roof. It didn't help the spasms at all, and it wasn't long before I booted it into touch.

Having had a break from Botox, I went back for another round and this time I asked the nurse to try to control my mouth movements as well as the eye twitches. Boy, did she control my mouth. The whole side of my face was frozen to the extent that I couldn't smile, laugh or project any sort of facial expression. I felt at one of my lowest ebbs after this treatment and the next 3 months were really tough. Gog would say 'Shall we go to………………………..' and I would freak on him, explaining that I didn't want to go anywhere. I recall my son's 30th birthday party where my ex husband brought his new 'girlfriend'. The feelings of being a lesser person than her in every respect still live with me, even though she had the personality of a dead dog. This should have been a fabulous family occasion, but for me it was an ordeal that I just wanted over and done with. That frozen, asymmetrical Botox face felt worse than the spasms, even though I looked years younger…… on one side.

I again went back to the doctor and this time 'the boy' agreed to a referral to the neurologist. After a few months wait I had an appointment with a neurologist in Southampton. As luck would have it, my spasms went into remission just before I saw him and so there I was in the neurology department trying to make my face spasm which it would not. The neurologist's opening remark to me was 'I see you've tried Carbamazepine and it made your blood pressure go up. Let me tell you that this cannot happen.' My opening line to the neurologist was 'So are you calling me a liar Doctor?' This wasn't a great start. He asked me a few questions about my spasms but said that he couldn't see anything wrong with me. He did a couple of tests, like making me walk in a straight line and getting me to point my finger at my nose and then encouraged me out of his office as fast as he could. He wrote to my GP basically saying that there was nothing wrong with me.

Gog and I got married in 2008. I insisted on not inviting anyone to the ceremony because I couldn't cope with the fuss or the photos and I didn't want my spasms to get worse with the stress of a wedding. I don't have a single photo of me in spasm mode; I became an accomplished camera dodger.

OK, now I was in remission again and I felt as if I had been given a clean bill of health. So, what did I do? Instead of cherishing the quiet face, I got a very well paid job where I was out of my depth. And you know what happened next, don't you? Yes, those old spasms came back with a ferocity that frightened me. I had been in remission for a full 8 months on this occasion and had dared to think that I was cured. Not so. I was now quite far up the creek without a paddle. Botox had failed, the job was too much for me, I was starting to spasm day and night and I was dizzy off and on when laying down. I've never been a good sleeper and have always been a bit of an over the counter junkie for anything which would make me sleep, but now I was starting to take as many pills as I could lay my hands on. Tiredness is HFS's accomplice and I needed to get some sleep. I moved out of the marital bed and relations with Gog were hitting an all-time low. I remember trying to kiss him and he was spasming nearly as much as me with the shock waves. This really wasn't the electricity that a couple needed!

I went to see another neurologist, but, just as before, my spasms weren't playing ball at the time. There was something about a white coat that made my spasms stop altogether. Weird. Anyway, he wasn't interested in sending me for an MRI scan and gave me the impression that he thought I was making it all up. Thanks doctor.

I was now 5 years into my HFS journey and I wasn't 'me' any more. There were times where I wanted Gog to leave me because then I wouldn't have to talk any more. In 2007 my middle son and his wife gave birth to my first grandchild which gave me joy that I couldn't have dreamed of, but it was still tough. I used to try to smile at darling Lulu and felt my face contorting as I did so. It wasn't long before baby Lulu was spasming back at me because babes will often imitate what they see. My eldest son was an Army pilot and was sent to Afghanistan in 2008. Can you imagine what that did to a neurotic wreck like me, not to mention him of course? I was spasming for England, Scotland, Wales and now Ireland too. I would spend every night awake worrying about my son and every day just trying to get through the twitchy day at work. In 2009 I had had enough and gave up work altogether; I had admitted defeat, with HFS winning.

I never exactly felt suicidal but I remember feeling that it would be no bad thing if I were to die, even though by now (2009) I had 5 grandchildren and everything to live for. I remember doing deals with God that if he would bring my son safely back from Afghanistan then he could have my life any time he wanted. Jesus clearly didn't want me for a sunbeam just yet.

Having given up work, I did feel some relief from my spasms, but they were ever present. I didn't like going to the shops and remember always trying to go at times when I wouldn't bump into anyone I knew. It was like being a criminal, trying to avoid the cops. I was by now wearing my sunglasses all the time, summer and winter. I must have looked a bit like one of the Mafia in our sleepy little English village. Gog is a big drinker and loves the pub, but he always had to drink alone. His life was being limited by HFS because the last thing I wanted to do was mix with people and have to talk to them in the pub. Drinking or eating in public were tough assignments for this HFS granny, so Gog was on his own. My condition was definitely impacting on my husband, but he was very good...... most of the time. Sometimes he got irritable that we never did anything or went anywhere any more, but he seldom complained.

Around 2009 I came across a site on the internet called the 'Hemifacial Spasm Association' (I think it's now dormant) and this site had a lot of useful information which made me feel less alone in my pity party. I noticed some good reports about a Professor in Bristol, UK and decided that, whatever the cost, I had to see this man. My daughter offered to pay for me to see him privately and so off I went to Bristol, about 100 miles away. I had an MRI scan and saw the Prof a few minutes later. He was so friendly and approachable, and, finally, I knew that someone understood this thing that had been blighting my life. He had a skeleton's head on his desk, with lots of little coloured wires representing the nerves that feed the face. He explained HFS to me, pointing at the head on the desk, and he compared it to electrical circuits which are touching one another and causing sparks/spasms. I think his explanation was a lot more technical than that but that's all I remembered. The 'Prof' looked at my MRI and said that I had a 'good channel' for operating within, whatever that meant. He offered me surgery right away at a cost of about £14,000. This was out of the question for me and I told him so. I didn't mention my little gambling habit which always kept me poor. Anyway, he was kind enough to recommend a neurosurgeon, who trained under him, and who operated from an NHS Hospital in Bristol. I felt as if I had won the lottery after leaving the Professor's office; it was sheer relief that at last someone had taken me seriously and believed that I had something wrong with me. I don't think I was seriously thinking about having surgery at this stage but it was fantastic to know that I had this option. Did I mention that I've always been a coward of the first order when it comes to operations?

The Professor wrote to my GP and, armed with this proper diagnosis, she was happy to refer me to the Bristol neurosurgeon. I waited around 6 months to see him but I wasn't disappointed. The Professor had recommended that I should take a video of my spasms in case they decided to do their 'white coat' thing when I saw the surgeon. The spasms and my heart nearly stopped when I saw the lovely, softly spoken neurosurgeon. He was a very tall, imposing man but was gentle in his manner. He listened carefully, looked at my MRI and just said 'This condition is emotionally blunting'. At this point I dissolved into uncontrollable tears. It was as if someone had unlocked an emotional valve in just a few words. Several tissues later the neurosurgeon offered me surgery on the NHS. I said 'yes' in a scared squeaky voice.

There was a 4 month wait for surgery and, as luck would have it, I developed a seriously painful shoulder condition during the waiting period. I hurt all the time and was put on some heavy meds to control the pain, but nothing really worked. Every movement was excruciating. All of a sudden HFS was deprioritised and getting rid of the pain was all I could think of. So, my HFS surgery was put off for a year whilst this shoulder condition either healed or needed surgery. Thankfully it healed but I was emotionally drained from it all, with 2012 being one of the worst periods in my life. The Neurosurgeon was patient with me and, against the rules, allowed me to remain on his waiting list, but always at the bottom. This was good really because I didn't have to confront the reality of having my head opened up.

During this anus horribilis I joined an HFS internet forum called Patient.co.uk. I met some incredible people on that site and one man in particular, who was a Chinese Singaporian called Leon. Leon held my virtual hand and gave me the confidence to move forward towards surgery for my HFS. He had had a failed MVD operation but still encouraged me to give it a go. I became a bit obsessive on the site, but gained so much from talking to others and realising that I wasn't alone. Leon also recommended me to the Facebook Hemifacial Spasm Support Group site and this opened up a whole world of information and new HFS friends. But I still wasn't sure that I would go through with the surgery because I was more or less convinced that I would die under the anaesthetic. With this in mind I rang my neurosurgeon and arranged a telephone consultation to ask him loads of probing questions about how many of these operations he had done, what his success rate was, how many people had died, how many had lost hearing etc. He was brilliant and answered my questions with total honesty. He told me that he expected me to be OK and this was what I needed to hear. I waited a further 4 months before my name came to the top of the neurosurgeon's list. It was by now 2013.

I went into extreme panic mode during the week before my scheduled surgery, but in the day or two before my admission to hospital I felt a strange and eerie calm, almost as if I was stepping into a parallel universe. I had updated my Will (nothing to leave except good wishes) and written notes to all my family in case I didn't come home again. My house was in order.

My family were all very supportive of me having the surgery, even though they must have been scared stiff for me. My brother in particular spurred me on and told me that I owed it to myself to try to get my old self back. He's a former headmaster and very strict, and I love him for his decisiveness. I think a lot of people had a personal agenda in wanting the old me back again and who could blame them?

Gog took me to the hospital on the day before surgery and I asked him to go home again. I tend to like to do difficult things on my own and people just annoy me if they start fussing. I only told Leon, my forum friend, that I was going for surgery and I asked if he would update the forum with my progress, should I come through the operation……..

I didn't sleep a wink in the hospital on the night before surgery and, in my upset and sleep deprived state I decided to run away from the hospital at about 5.00 am. Sadly Gog had left me with no clothes and no money and so a 100 mile streak was going to be a tad embarrassing. The lady in the next bed, whom I told that I intended to run, was a lovely but very firm Welsh dragon. She gave me a stiff talking to and simply said 'You wouldn't 'ave come 'ere if you didn't want to be cured'. The next ogre I came across was the Chinese nurse who was sent over to counsel me out of my sobbing state. Chinese counselling is nothing like English counselling. She marched over to me and said 'Stop this now. Get in the shower and put your stockings on'. Her complete lack of compassion was the right approach and shocked me into submission.

It wasn't long before a certain teenage-looking doctor came to see me to do the final checks for anaesthetic. When I saw how young he was I was pretty certain that I had seen my last day dawning. Another doctor came to 'consent me' and I told him that I didn't want him to spell out all the risks again, I knew them all too well. He was very good and just let me sign the form.

Thankfully I was first on the neurosurgeon's list that day and so I didn't have any further opportunity for second thoughts before they bundled me onto the trolley and into a store cupboard which turned out to be the anaesthetic room. A few wires on the chest, a canula in my hand, a mask over my face and 'goodnight Angela'. It was 20 June 2013 and I was 62 years of age. The big question was 'Would I make 63?'

Much to my surprise I woke up alive and still 'on earth'. The neurosurgeon had shaken my hand before the operation and told me that he would do nothing to endanger my life. The lovely man was reading me like a book and had sussed just how scared and neurotic I was; he knew all the right buttons to press, in the nicest possible way. I woke up in the Recovery Room insisting that I had not had the operation because I felt perfectly fine. The nurse advised me that I had had surgery and that as I was waking up I had been babbling extensively about the young anaesthetist; I doubt that it was very complimentary.

I didn't need to go into ICU (Intensive Care Unit) and was back on the ward 4.5 hours after going down. My first thought was to text Gog and ring my daughter. They couldn't believe that I was well enough to do this and didn't realise that I was as high as a kite on steroids. Apparently I was slurring my speech like an old soak. My next thought was to get something to eat; I love food and hadn't had any for hours. I had a full lunch and then vomited it up in its entirety an hour later. I didn't give a damn, I was alive.

The neurosurgeon came to see me at about 4.00 pm and told me that, although the operation had gone well, he wasn't sure that he had fixed the problem because it would have been too dangerous to go deeper into the brain stem where an artery was pressing on the facial nerve. I honestly didn't care that I wasn't fixed, I was so relieved to still be here. I can't tell you how proud I was of myself for going through with the operation and it was almost worth it to have the lovely surgeon at my bedside. Does everyone fall in love with their surgeon I wonder? Later that day I started spasming quite badly but I didn't care. My attitude was that I had no right to be cured and that any improvement would be a bonus.

I felt a bit dizzy but was able to mobilise like a 90 year old within a couple of hours of the surgery. I had the anti-sickness meds and anti-clotting injections into my tummy, plus any painkillers I could lay my hands on. I continued with the steroids which had also been given during surgery. My only real side effect of the surgery was a very sore eye which needed antibiotic cream and cooling pads. The wound began to tighten a bit but was never very painful.

I stayed in hospital for 4 days and had visits from my faithful Gog and my lovely son and daughter who both seemed to love me just that little bit more than before the op. Their relief and love was tangible. Meanwhile, I continued to have spasms but they didn't get me down.
The nursing was usually very good at the hospital, but occasionally quite bad. As a rule it was the day staff who were excellent and the night staff who seemed to be a bit 'off piste'. One night I had a bad headache and so I got up and asked the Chinese nurse 'Can I have some drugs?' I thought she was about to produce a flick knife when she responded 'What you mean drugs?' Eventually I reassured her that I was not doing a hold up on the morphine stash and that I simply wanted some painkillers. She was actually a very good nurse but we had some communication difficulties. On another night there were some nurses who appeared to be of African origin who insisted on giving each patient every drug on their drug chart. It was meant to be 'as required' but they weren't having any of this. I was assertive in refusing what I didn't want but the lady opposite me gave in to their insistence and was out cold for 24 hours afterwards. Sorry if this makes me sound like a racist; I don't think I am, but I do think communication can sometimes be challenging between different nationalities and cultures.

I was relieved to leave hospital and to be heading home to my lovely, dark, quiet bedroom. In only 4 days I had become quite institutionalised and I felt like an escaping prisoner on the journey home. I had an anti-sickness tablet and, with the help of a comfy pillow, the drive home was perfectly OK. The countryside looked greener, the air smelled sweeter and I felt like a super hero. Yes, what a drama queen I am.

I was very kind to myself during the next few weeks of my recovery. I came down a bit when the steroids were stopped and gave in to having regular daily sleeps and no more visitors than I really wanted. I didn't feel like reading or watching the television, and just wallowed in my comfy bed, making guest appearances downstairs from time to time. I took painkillers for a low, dull headache and it was all very bearable. I had the 20 staples out and washed my hair on day 6 post surgery. It was a bit scary to have the dressing removed and to see my wound for the first time, but I got Gog to take a photo so that I could revel in my bravery. Some days I did too much, like going for a long walk and then nursing my arm all the way home, but generally I did what the doctor ordered and let Gog and the family look after me. I recall that crossing the road felt a bit unsafe because I couldn't swing my neck as easily as before. What an irony it would have been to have been knocked down after all that bother.

I have to say that this was the first time in my life that I have just given in and been looked after by others and I loved every minute of it. I was a geriatric Prima Dona and I switched off the world for a few weeks. Cards and flowers arrived in abundance and our home looked like a funeral parlour. After about 3 weeks I felt loads better but my neck was still a bit too rigid to feel confident in driving. I am not sure that, if I had still been working, I would have gone back until at least 8 weeks post op. This was when I began to feel strong again, but I still felt tired a lot of the time. The spasms continued but not as aggressively as before and not in the night.

Six weeks was a major milestone for me because I started to drive again and my spasms suddenly stopped happening. This literally happened overnight and at first I couldn't believe it, but they have never reappeared. I have my fingers and knickers crossed as I say this.
I am now 6 years post op and have had no further spasms. Occasionally, when tired or stressed, I get a little flutter, sometimes in both eyes, but I refuse to think that HFS is returning. The neurosurgeon gave me my life back and I shall remain eternally grateful. I continue to contribute to the Facebook and Patient forums online and the people I've met (well, not met, actually) have enriched my life in ways that I didn't think possible. I love life with my 6 grandchildren, and Gog and I have a normal relationship again. We go to the pub, go on holiday and we enjoy our families. I do still find social gatherings a bit too much and I suspect this will be permanent now. It takes a long time to withdraw from society and a long time to reintegrate too. I have thought about going back to work, but, there again……………….. I don't think so. My daughter got married in 2019 and it was so good to embrace the camera rather than dodging it; we have some lovely photos which I shall always treasure just a little more than I would have done.

I hope my story might help others to realise that they are not alone with this thing which punches well above its weight in terms of its impact on everyday life. We don't all have the option of surgery but there is always support online for you, wherever or whoever you may be. Don't give up and don't be as big a coward as me.

Cindy Teta

My name is Cindy Teta. I am 64 years old and live in Pennsylvania. This is my Hemifacial Spasm Story.

My HFS Journey began May 27, 2010. I awoke on my 55th birthday with a slight twitch on my lower eyelid. I thought the twitch would eventually stop, but instead it progressed to my cheek and mouth. I began researching and was sure I had Hemifacial Spasms. In October 2010 I was seen by my General Practitioner (GP) and she confirmed HFS. She recommended six months to check progression.

In April 2011, my GP ordered an MRI to rule out MS, Tumor, etc. The MRI read negative by a Radiologist. She referred me to a Neurologist but, after extensive research, I decided to wait because I wasn't ready to try Botox or medication.

In July 2013 I took a six month leave of absence from my employment to care for my bedridden Father. My HFS stopped for the entire six months only to return with vengeance. I did not return to my 41-year profession, as I was one-on-one and not in a comfortable position, having HFS, to continue my career.

I continued research and found information on MVD and the Jannetta Procedure. I had read that HFS was first identified in the 1800's, but it wasn't until the 1960's when Neurosurgeon Dr. Peter Jannetta did the first keyhole surgery, which was named the "Jannetta Procedure".

In spring of 2017 my spasms were unbearable and I returned to my GP only to be discouraged to consider MVD. I was again referred to a Neurologist for Botox. I called a Neurosurgeon expert in HFS and MVD surgery and took the first available appointment for tests and a consult. On June 15, 2017, I had all the tests and the Neurosurgeon consult done in one day. The 3D MRI of the vascular structure confirmed arterial compressions along the attached segment of the facial nerve by the vertebral artery. I elected to undergo surgery. My daughter was two months into Chemotherapy so I scheduled my MVD four months from confirming MVD for HFS.

On October 20, 2017, my Neurosurgeon padded two areas and did a Gore-Tex sling of the artery with TachoSil adhesive to the Dura of my brain. After a one hour, forty-five-minute surgery I awoke in recovery and was transferred to the ICU for three nights. I was spasm free for only two days. I did vomit nonstop for 48 hours and ate very little. One day post op I had Shingles on the opposite side of MVD, which was diagnosed by my GP six days post MVD. One hundred seventeen pills were added to my recovery, not including the Oxycodone script that I refused. I had been exposed to someone that had the live Shingles virus vaccine 17 days prior to my MVD so it was not related to the surgery. I had no hearing loss or dizziness. I had no pain except a headache and I had full neck motion so I was able to drive day seven post MVD. My worst head pain occurred during weeks seven and eight.

After hospital discharge I only used Tylenol until I started my Shingles medication. I did not return to work for eight weeks and, once returning, I worked a maximum of twenty hours per week until six months post MVD. My work is physical and my full tonus spasms (including contracted facial muscle up to one minute and eye closure) are unbearable and exhausting. I continue to be hopeful and open to another surgery. I have full tonus spasms with very few moments of calm in addition to Tinnitus off and on. I had another MRI and a Neurosurgeon consultation on June 20, 2019 with the same doctor who did my MVD. Per him, he can go in and massage the nerve with a 50% chance of improvement, but increased risk including a greater chance of hearing loss. My Neurosurgeon advised against another MVD. He stated that I had severe compressions pre MVD, which I am assuming may have caused nerve damage.

I have never tried Botox or medications for my HFS, but might consider Botox since my spasms are almost 24/7 with little relief. I have always lived a healthy lifestyle and tried everything possible to control HFS to no avail. In my opinion, MVD is the only possible cure. HFS is embarrassing, depressing, exhausting and a horrid condition. Hopefully I will be free of HFS someday! I know members of my support group have become spasm free as far out as 3 ½ years so I will not give up hope!

Glossary

BEB – Abbreviation for Benign Essential Blepharospasm.

Benign Essential Blepharospasm – A type of dystonia causing abnormal blinking and/or spasms of the eyelids. This condition can cause what is referred to as functional blindness in an individual.

Blepharospasm – Abnormal blinking and/or spasms of the eyelids. It is often secondary caused by another medical condition. If not, it may be Benign Essential Blepharospasm.

EMG – Abbreviation for Electromyography. A test using needles (electrodes) by inserting into various muscles. It's used to detect neurological abnormalities.

Hemifacial Spasm – A neurological condition causing one side of the face to twitch or spasm involuntary. It can be caused by various reasons. The most common cause is a compression of the facial nerve by a blood vessel or artery. Although rare, it can also occur bi-lateral.

HFS – Abbreviation for Hemifacial Spasm.

Microvascular Decompression Surgery – Considered as a type of brain surgery where a compressed cranial nerve is located and Teflon sponges are inserted to separate the nerve and the offending artery/vessel.

MRA (Brain) – Abbreviation for Magnetic Resonance Angiography. This is another type of MRI of the brain that is considered better than a standard MRI.

MRI (Brain) – Abbreviation for Magnetic Resonance Imaging. This test produces detail images of the brain.

MVD – Abbreviation for Microvascular Decompression Surgery.

Bravery

It takes bravery every day to face the world with this condition.

It takes bravery to face Botox.

It takes bravery to face major surgery.

It takes bravery to face the fact that same surgery may not be successful and you're back to square one facing it all over again.

It takes bravery to be us.

Kim Marie Puckett
Auckland, New Zealand

www.ingramcontent.com/pod-product-compliance
Lightning Source LLC
Chambersburg PA
CBHW081457220526
45466CB00008B/2687